100 Questions & Answers About Cancer Symptoms and Cancer Treatment Side Effects

Joanne Frankel Kelvin,
RN, MSN, AOCN
Memorial Sloan-Kettering Cancer Center

Leslie B. Tyson,
MS, APN-BC, OCN
Memorial Sloan-Kettering Cancer Center

JONES AND BARTLETT PUBLISHERS
Sudbury, Massachusetts
BOSTON   TORONTO   LONDON   SINGAPORE

World Headquarters
Jones and Bartlett
Publishers
40 Tall Pine Drive
Sudbury, MA 01776
info@jbpub.com
www.jbpub.com

Jones and Bartlett
Publishers Canada
2406 Nikanna Road
Mississauga, ON L5C 2W6
CANADA

Jones and Bartlett
Publishers International
Barb House, Barb Mews
London W6 7PA
UK

Library of Congress Cataloging-in-Publication Data
Kelvin, Joanne Frankel.
  100 questions & answers about cancer symptoms and cancer treatment side effects / Joanne Frankel
Kelvin, Leslie B. Tyson.
    p. cm.
Includes index.
  ISBN 0-7637-2612-5 (pbk.)
  1. Cancer--Popular works. 2. Cancer--Treatment--Complications--Popular works. 3.
Antineoplastic agents--Side effects--Popular works. I. Title: One hundred questions and answers
about cancer symptoms and cancer treatment side effects. II. Tyson, Leslie B. III. Title.
  RC263.K44 2004
                                2004002748

Production Credits:
Chief Executive Officer: Clayton Jones
Chief Operating Officer: Don W. Jones, Jr.
Executive V.P. & Publisher: Robert W. Holland, Jr.
V.P., Sales and Marketing: William J. Kane
V.P., Design and Production: Anne Spencer
V.P., Manufacturing and Inventory Control: Therese Bräuer
Executive Publisher: Christopher Davis
Special Projects Editor: Elizabeth Platt
Editorial Assistant: Kathy Richardson
Senior Marketing Manager: Alisha Weisman
Marketing Associate: Matthew Payne
Cover Design: Philip Regan/Bret Kerr
Cover Image: "Jestina's Garden" 1996. © Hyacinth Manning/Superstock
Printing and Binding: Malloy, Inc.
Cover Printing: Malloy, Inc.

Printed in the United States of America
08 07 06 05 04 10 9 8 7 6 5 4 3 2

CONTENTS

A diagnosis of cancer presents numerous challenges. Initially, you must learn about the disease, select the physicians who will care for you, and decide on what treatment to receive, if choices are offered to you. Then, you must focus on coping with the day-to-day problems you may encounter.

We hope that this book will provide information and support to help you in meeting these challenges, from your initial diagnosis, through your treatment, and after your treatment is completed. We have included information about cancer and cancer treatment, but the focus is on managing the symptoms of the disease and side effects of treatment. Equally important is information we hope will help you and your family cope with the emotional and practical concerns that will come up during your treatment. We are grateful to Jones and Bartlett for recognizing the need to offer a book such as this to people with cancer.

Joanne Frankel Kelvin is an oncology nurse at Memorial Sloan-Kettering Cancer Center, currently working as the Nurse Leader in the Department of Radiation Oncology. She has been a nurse for 28 years, specializing in oncology nursing for most of that time. She has been inspired by the courage and strength of her patients and their families. She dedicates this book to them with gratitude for all they have taught her over the years. In addition, she thanks her husband for his constant support.

Leslie B. Tyson, MS, APN-BC, OCN is a nurse practitioner at Memorial Sloan-Kettering Cancer Center; she currently works on the Thoracic Oncology Service. She has been an oncology nurse for 27 years and has worked at the Center for the same length of time. She dedicates this book to all of her patients for all they have taught her over the years and to her husband, Gary S. Rudolph, for all his support and encouragement.

PART ONE

Cancer and Cancer Treatment

What is cancer?

Why does cancer cause symptoms?

What are the treatments for cancer?

More . . .

1. What is cancer?

A cancer is generally named for the organ or type of cell in which it began to grow.

Cancer is a term used to describe over 100 different diseases that have certain features in common. It begins with a change in the structure and function of a particular cell that causes it to divide without control; it can subsequently invade and damage surrounding tissues, and cells can break away and spread to distant areas in the body. A cancer is generally named for the organ or type of cell in which it began to grow.

Cancers are generally classified as solid tumors and liquid tumors. Solid tumors begin in a particular organ of the body, for example, breast cancer or lung cancer. Liquid tumors begin in the bone marrow or lymph system of the body. These include leukemia, lymphoma, and multiple myeloma.

Tumor

an abnormal swelling or mass.

Benign

a non-cancerous tumor.

Malignant

a cancerous tumor; can invade surrounding structures and spread to a distant site.

Grade

a measure of how abnormal a cell appears when examined under a microscope; in some cases predicts how aggressive the cancer.

Stage

a measure of how extensive the cancer is, how much it has spread.

Different terms are often used in speaking about cancer; understanding these will be helpful when you speak with your doctor or read information about your cancer. A **tumor** is any mass or swelling in the body. Looking at a sample of the tumor cells under a microscope is necessary to determine if it is a **benign** (noncancerous) tumor or a **malignant** (cancerous) tumor. The **grade** of the tumor is also determined by the microscopic examination. This describes the appearance of the cells, which often indicates how aggressive the cancer is. The **stage** or extent of disease describes if the cancer has spread to other parts of the body. A variety of tests is needed to determine the stage, for example blood tests, computed tomography (CT), magnetic resonance imaging (MRI), radionuclide scanning, positron emission tomography (PET), and, in some types of cancer, samples of bone marrow. There are four stages for most types of cancer. These are generally defined as follows. Stage I means the tumor is localized to a small area within the organ in which it started. Stage II means the cancer has spread to lymph nodes in the area. Stage III means the tumor is **locally advanced** (invaded surrounding structures). Stage IV means the tumor has **metastasized** (spread to a distant area in the body).

Locally advanced
describes when a cancerous tumor has spread to surrounding structures.

Metastasized
describes when a cancerous tumor has spread to a distant site, for example the bones, the liver, or the brain.

2. Why does cancer cause symptoms?

The symptoms of cancer depend on where the cancer begins and how it grows. If the tumor is close to the surface of the body, one may see a lump or swelling, a change in color of the skin or mucous membranes, a sore that doesn't heal, or bleeding. If the tumor is deep within the body, symptoms may not develop until the tumor grows large enough to press on other structures. This may block one of the passageways of the body, causing obstruction. For example, blockage of an airway in the lung can cause a cough, blockage of the intestine can cause constipation or vomiting, and blockage of the bile duct can cause jaundice. As tumors grow they can cause pain from pressure on different parts of the body and may cause fluid to accumulate within the body. Fluid in the abdominal cavity is called **ascites**; this can cause swelling of the belly and pain. Fluid in the chest is called a **pleural effusion**; this can cause cough and shortness of breath. Symptoms may not develop until the cancer has metastasized. For example, spread to the liver can cause abnormal blood tests, pain, and jaundice; spread to the bone can cause pain; and spread to the brain can cause confusion. Having cancer may also change certain aspects of the body's metabolism; this can cause weight loss, fever, sweats, or fatigue.

Ascites
abnormal build up of fluid in the abdominal cavity.

Pleural effusion
abnormal build up of fluid in the chest cavity.

Cancer and Cancer Treatment

3. *What are the treatments for cancer?*

Cancer treatments include

- Surgery to remove the tumor, sometimes with surrounding tissue and local **lymph nodes**. Surgery can also be done to remove part of a tumor or to relieve symptoms caused by the tumor.
- Radiation therapy, the use of high-energy radiation to destroy or shrink the tumor (see Question 4).
- Chemotherapy, drugs that destroy cancer cells (see Question 5).
- Hormonal therapy, alteration of the hormone levels in the body to slow or stop the growth of certain cancer cells (see Question 7).
- Biologic therapy to stimulate the immune system to fight off cancer (see Question 8).

Surgery and radiation therapy are local treatments, directed to a particular part of the body. Chemotherapy, hormonal therapy, and biologic therapy are systemic treatments, which travel through the bloodstream to all parts of the body.

Cancer treatments are constantly evolving as we better understand the biology of how cancers develop and grow and as we develop new technologies to perform less invasive surgery and to more precisely deliver radiation therapy. For many cancers, combined modality therapy, a combination of treatments, is used.

For many cancers, a combination of treatments is used.

Oncologists, doctors who specialize in the treatment of cancer, will recommend the type of treatment that is best for you. This will depend on the type of cancer, the stage of disease, and your general state of health. Depending on your situation, the goal of treatment may be to cure the disease, to control the growth of the cancer, or to relieve symptoms you may have (**palliation**).

4. What is radiation therapy and how is it given?

Radiation therapy treats disease with high energy in the form of waves or particles. As the energy passes through the body, it damages the cells in its path, destroying the cancer cells or shrinking the tumor. Normal cells in the path of the energy are also affected by this energy; however, normal cells are better able to recover from the effects of radiation than cancer cells. Radiation therapy is carefully planned to ensure an accurate dose is delivered to the tumor site while minimizing the dose received by the surrounding normal tissues.

Radiation therapy is most commonly administered as external beam treatment. Beams of radiation are directed from a machine, such as a **linear accelerator**, to a particular part of the body. Before beginning treatment, a simulation is scheduled to begin the planning process. You are positioned on a table as you will be lying each day for treatment. Special immobilizing devices such as face masks, molds, or cradles may be made to ensure the position is correct each day. Skin markings, usually in the form of permanent tattoos the size of a pinhead, are made; these are also used to position you correctly each day. Images are taken to localize the area to be treated. Depending on the treatment planned, these may be done using x-rays, CTs, MRIs, or PETs. The radiation oncologist, with a physicist and **dosimetrist**, will then decide on the number of radiation beams, at what angles they should be directed, and how they should be shaped.

Palliation
treatment aimed at relieving physical, emotional, social, and spiritual symptoms to improve quality of life.

Radiation therapy
the use of high-energy radiation to destroy cancer cells; also called radiotherapy or irradiation.

Radiation therapy is carefully planned to ensure an accurate dose is delivered to the tumor site while minimizing the dose received by the surrounding normal tissues.

Cancer and Cancer Treatment

5

Once the planning is completed and the radiation oncologist confirms that the dose being delivered to the tumor site is correct and will not cause excessive side effects, treatment begins. Treatment generally does not require hospitalization. It is given every day, Monday through Friday, until the total dose has been delivered. This generally takes anywhere from 2 to 8 weeks, depending on the disease being treated. People are generally in the treatment room anywhere from 15 to 30 minutes. Radiation therapists will position you correctly and then leave the room. Using controls outside of the room, they turn on the beam; these are on for only 1 to 5 minutes. There is no sensation at all when the beam is on; there is no pain, burning, or discomfort. You will see the treatment machine move around you to the different positions needed to deliver each beam, and you will hear the machine as it turns on and off.

During treatment with external beam radiation therapy, you will be seen weekly by your radiation oncologist and radiation oncology nurse. They will evaluate how you are tolerating the treatment and help you to manage any side effects you develop.

Brachytherapy

radiation treatment that involves the placement of sealed radioactive material (for example, seeds or wires) into the body where they emit radiation as they decay (break down); also called implants or internal radiation.

Radiation therapy can also be administered with internal treatment. One form of internal radiation is called **brachytherapy**, in which a radioactive source in the form of a seed, ribbon, or tube is positioned inside the body. Depending on the type of source used, it may be kept in place for a number of minutes or for several days. Some sources are left in place permanently and are referred to as implants. While the implant is in place, it emits radiation to the tissues in the immediate surrounding area. Permanent implants decay and lose their energy over time, usually a number of months.

The other form of internal radiation uses radioactive material taken by mouth or injected into a vein. This travels through the body and tends to collect where tumor cells are located. It emits radiation until it is eliminated by the body. Internal radiation often requires hospitalization, and some forms also require isolation for a period of time because of the radiation being emitted from your body while the source is in place. Your radiation oncologist and a physicist from the radiation safety service will review any precautions you need to take.

Many advances in radiation therapy have been made in recent years. Technological advances, such as three-dimensional conformal radiation therapy, intensity-modulated radiation therapy, intraoperative radiation, and stereotactic radiosurgery, are aimed at getting more precision in the delivery of the radiation beam while reducing the doses received by the surrounding normal tissues. Biologic advances are based on our increasing knowledge of how cancers grow. They include the use of concurrent chemotherapy and hyperfractionated treatment, in which treatment is given in smaller doses more than once a day.

For additional information on radiation therapy, read *Radiation Therapy and You: A Guide to Self-Help During Cancer Treatment*, available at *www.cancer.gov* or 800-4-CANCER.

5. What is chemotherapy and how is it given?

Chemotherapy is the treatment of cancer with drugs that destroy cancer cells. Chemotherapy can also damage normal (healthy) cells, especially healthy cells in

Chemotherapy
treatment with drugs that destroy cancer cells or stop them from growing.

the lining of the mouth, the bone marrow, gastrointestinal tract, and hair follicles. Damage to healthy cells is the reason that chemotherapy causes side effects (see Question 12). Cancer cells cannot repair the damage caused by chemotherapy, and they eventually die. However, healthy cells can usually repair the damage caused by chemotherapy.

There are more than 200 different types of cancer and over 50 different chemotherapy drugs available.

There are more than 200 different types of cancer and over 50 different chemotherapy drugs available. Your doctor will decide what type of chemotherapy is right for you, based on where your cancer started, if it has metastasized (spread) to other areas of your body, and how healthy you are. For many types of cancer, a combination of drugs is used to increase the number of cells destroyed.

Chemotherapy can be given with the goal of curing cancer, controlling the disease, or relieving symptoms (palliation). Primary or **neoadjuvant chemotherapy** is given before surgery; given in this way, the chemotherapy is used to shrink the tumor and make it easier for the surgeon to remove. Chemotherapy may also be given in this way before radiation therapy. **Adjuvant chemotherapy** is given after surgery if there is a risk that microscopic cancer cells (those that are unable to be seen) are left behind after surgery. In people with metastatic cancer, which usually cannot be cured, chemotherapy can extend life and relieve symptoms.

Neoadjuvant chemotherapy

treatment with chemotherapy before the primary treatment, for example before surgery; often used to shrink the tumor.

Adjuvant chemotherapy

treatment used after a tumor has been removed surgically to destroy any remaining cancer cells.

Chemotherapy can be given in any form that other drugs are given. It is most commonly given intravenously (IV), through a thin needle inserted into a vein; the needle is taken out after the treatment is completed. Sometimes a special thin flexible catheter is placed in a large vein in the body and left in place over a number of months or years, until it is no longer needed. This avoids having to stick your vein with a needle for each treatment. (See Question 6 for more information about these catheters.) When giving chemotherapy intravenously, it can be pushed in quickly (over minutes), dripped in over a number of hours, or even infused continuously over a number of days. For some types of cancer, chemotherapy is given into an artery rather than a vein.

Chemotherapy can also be injected under the skin (subcutaneously), into the muscle, or into the cerebrospinal fluid; for some types of cancer, it is instilled into a body cavity (for example, the bladder or the abdomen). For some types of skin cancer, chemotherapy can be applied as a cream or ointment directly to the skin.

There is increasing use of chemotherapy that can be given orally (by mouth). It may be in the form of a tablet, capsule, or liquid. Patients commonly take oral chemotherapy themselves at home. If you are responsible for administering your own chemotherapy, it is important to take it exactly as prescribed. If you are unable to do this, you need to notify your doctor immediately. Ask your doctor or nurse if there are any special instructions to follow when handling chemotherapy at home.

Chemotherapy is given according to a particular schedule that is based on the type of cancer being treated and the particular drugs being used. It may be given daily, weekly, every 2 to 3 weeks, or monthly. The schedule is often described as being in "cycles," with treatment given for a defined period followed by a rest to allow the normal tissues of the body to recover from the effects of the chemotherapy. The chemotherapy may be given for a specific period of time (for example, six cycles) or may be given indefinitely.

Diagnostic tests will be ordered periodically during treatment with chemotherapy to evaluate how you are responding to treatment. Some tests evaluate how the tumor is responding; for example, a CT or MRI or bone scan may be ordered every 3 to 6 months to see if the tumor has gotten smaller, remained stable, or grown. Some tests evaluate how the normal tissues in your body are responding to treatment, to ensure the side effects of treatment are not putting you at risk for further problems. For example, before each treatment, a **complete blood count (CBC)** may be ordered to check that your blood counts are not too low (see Question 35) or blood chemistries (see Question 79) may be ordered to make sure your kidneys and liver are functioning normally.

Complete blood count (CBC)

a blood test to measure the number of white blood cells, red blood cells, and platelets.

6. What are vascular access devices? Do I need one?

Receiving treatment for cancer often requires the nurse to frequently access your veins to draw blood, administer chemotherapy, or give intravenous fluids. This is most commonly done by inserting a small metal or plastic needle under the skin into a vein in your hand or arm. Some people have veins that are difficult to find, and some people have veins that are very fragile. This may make visits to the doctor stressful, worrying if the nurse will be able to get into your vein. In addition, some chemotherapy drugs are very irritating or must be given over many hours or days, with a risk that the drug can leak out of the vein and seep under your skin. To counteract these problems, special long-term vascular access devices have been developed to make it easier and safer for you to receive your treatment. These devices all have a special thin flexible catheter or tube that is placed under the skin and inserted into a large vein in your chest, leading to your heart. The catheter may be left in place for a number of months or years, until it is no longer needed.

Special long-term vascular access devices have been developed to make it easier and safer for you to receive your treatment.

In one type of device, the catheter is attached to an "implantable port," a hollow round disk about the size of a quarter and a half inch high. This is placed under the skin, usually on the chest wall, under the collarbone. To access the device, the nurse inserts a special needle through the skin into the port. Between treatments a nurse must flush the device once a month to prevent it from clotting, but no other care is required. If you are "needle phobic," ask your nurse about EMLA cream. EMLA is a **topical anesthetic** that can be applied directly over the port; it will eliminate or reduce the pain of the needlestick. EMLA cream should be applied about 1 hour before your port is accessed.

Topical anesthetic medication applied to the surface of the body (for example the skin or mucous membranes) to numb the area.

In another type of device, the catheter exits through the skin and is called an "external catheter." Hickman catheters and PICC lines are examples of external catheters. The catheter may exit on the chest wall under the collarbone or on the arm. External catheters require frequent flushing and must be covered with a dressing. If you have an external catheter, your nurse will teach you how to take care of it. If your doctor feels you need a long-term catheter, he or she will recommend the type that is best for you.

Cancer and Cancer Treatment

These catheters all have the potential to become infected and develop blood clots. Call your doctor immediately if you develop redness, swelling, discharge, or pain at the site of the port or where the catheter exits the skin or if you develop swelling in the arm on the side of the catheter.

7. What types of hormonal therapies are used to treat cancer?

Hormones are chemicals produced by certain types of glands in the body. Cancer of the prostate and some cancers of the breast are stimulated by particular types of hormones. The cancer cells have receptors on their surface; the hormones bind to these receptors and stimulate the cells to multiply, causing the cancer to grow. **Hormonal therapies** are used to stop the body from producing these hormones or to block the activity of the hormones. The goal is to stop the cancer cells from dividing or to destroy them.

Prostate cancer is stimulated to grow by the male hormone testosterone, produced primarily by the testicles. Hormonal therapy is one treatment for prostate cancer. Some medications, for example, leuprolide and goserelin, stop the production of testosterone by the testicles. These are given by injection, usually once a month or every 3 months. This eliminates most of the testosterone in the body. Oral medication (for example, flutamide, bicalutamide) may be given in addition to the injections to block the receptors on the prostate cancer cells, inactivating any remaining testosterone that is circulating. Alternatively, men may have their testicles surgically removed (orchiectomy) to prevent testosterone production or may be given female hormones

Hormonal therapy
treatment that alters specific hormone levels in the body by stopping the production of the hormone, blocking the hormone, or adding hormone.

(for example, diethylstilbestrol) to counteract the effects of testosterone. Side effects of hormonal therapy in men with prostate cancer may include hot flashes, breast swelling and tenderness, decreased sex drive, inability to have an erection, weight gain, and fatigue.

Some types of breast cancer are stimulated to grow by the female hormone estrogen, produced primarily by the ovaries. Hormonal therapy is one treatment for breast cancer. The most commonly used medication is tamoxifen, which blocks the receptors on the breast cancer cells. Tamoxifen is an oral medication; other similar oral medications are being investigated. Fulvestrant is given by injection once a month; it not only blocks the receptors, it also destroys them. In women who have gone through menopause, the body still produces a small amount of estrogen; a group of drugs called aromatase inhibitors (for example, anastrozole, letrozole, exemestane) blocks the enzyme that stimulates this. Alternatively, women may receive leuprolide injections to stop the production of estrogen by the ovaries, may have their ovaries surgically removed, or may be given the hormone megestrol. Side effects of hormonal therapy in women with breast cancer may include hot flashes, vaginal discharge or irritation, fatigue, visual changes, and an increased risk of developing endometrial cancer or ovarian cysts.

8. What types of biologic therapies are used to treat cancer?

Biologic therapy, also called biotherapy or immunotherapy, includes a wide variety of approaches that use the immune system to treat cancer. The immune system consists of special cells and chemicals that have the ability to recognize and destroy foreign or abnormal cells,

Biologic therapy
treatment to stimulate the immune system to destroy cancer cells or strengthen the ability of the immune system to destroy the cancer cells.

13

including cancer cells. Biologic therapy introduces man-made immune substances into the body. These substances can destroy the cancer cells, make the cells more vulnerable to being destroyed by the body's own immune system, or strengthen the ability of the immune system to destroy the cancer cells. Most biologic therapies are still experimental. They include the following:

- Monoclonal antibodies: These antibodies are produced to recognize a specific abnormal protein on the surface of cancer cells. They can travel directly to these cells and attack them. Alternatively, they may be linked to chemotherapy or **radioactive isotopes** and carry these to the site of cancer; the chemotherapy or radioactive isotopes can then act to destroy the cancer cells. Because of their ability to differentiate between cancer cells and normal cells, monoclonal antibodies are a type of targeted therapy (see Question 9). Examples of monoclonal antibodies used in cancer treatment are rituximab, trastuzumab, gemtuzumab, and alemtuzumab. An example of a monoclonal antibody linked to a radioactive isotope is ibritumomab tiuxetan.
- Cytokines: These are chemicals that can attack cancer cells or stimulate the immune system. Examples of cytokines used in cancer treatment include interferon, interleukin, tumor necrosis factor, and colony-stimulating growth factors.
- Vaccines: These are made from cancer cells that have been inactivated. Vaccines stimulate the immune system to make antibodies to destroy the cancer cells in the body.

Radioactive isotopes

unstable elements that emit radioactivity as they decay (break down); used to take diagnostic images or to treat cancer.

9. What is targeted therapy?

In recent years, laboratory research has helped us gain a new understanding of the complex biologic pathways in the cell that cause cancers to develop, grow, and spread in the body. Targeted therapy works by blocking specific biologic pathways.

One example of a pathway that may be blocked by targeted therapy involves EGFR (**epidermal growth factor receptor**). This is a family of protein receptors seen in many cancer cells. When these receptors are stimulated, they send signals that activate a series of chemical reactions in the cell. These may cause the cancer cells to begin dividing and multiplying without control. The signals may also block the ability of the body to naturally destroy cells that are old, damaged, or mutated, including cancer cells. They may increase the formation of blood vessels that bring oxygen and nutrients to the cancer cells, enabling them to grow. Also, they may facilitate the ability of the cancer cells to invade surrounding tissues and spread to distant sites. The receptor sites and all these chemical reactions present possible targets for cancer treatment. The benefit of targeted therapy is that treatment will affect only the cancer cells, having minimal effect on the normal cells of the body. The challenge of future research will be to find the right targets. Examples of targeted therapy include gefitinib and imatinib.

10. What are clinical trials?

Pete's comment:

I felt initially that one of the advantages of getting treatment at a cancer center was the potential of participating in a clinical research study. Every day you hear about new drugs that may have a positive effect on cancer and I felt that participating in a trial was a good opportunity to take advantage of the newest scientific research. When my treat-

---

Targeted therapy works by blocking specific biologic pathways.

Epidermal growth factor (EGF) receptor

protein found on the surface of some cells; when EGF binds to the protein receptor it stimulates the cell to divide.

Targeted therapy treatment affects only the cancer cells, having minimal effect on the normal cells of the body.

Cancer and Cancer Treatment

15

ment options included a clinical trial, I didn't hesitate to participate.

Clinical trials are research studies designed to test new treatments on humans. Any kind of treatment may be studied. This includes methods of administering radiation therapy, drugs (including chemotherapy), biologic agents, nutritional therapies, medical devices, or even behavioral therapies. A single new treatment may be studied, or standard treatments combined in new ways may be studied.

New treatments are usually first developed in a laboratory and then tested in animals. If they seem to provide some benefit, they are tested in phases in humans to determine their safety and effectiveness.

- Phase I clinical trials are undertaken first, to determine the appropriate dose and schedule for the treatment and to determine the side effects of the treatment.
- Phase II clinical trials test the treatment on patients with a particular type of cancer to determine how effective the treatment is.
- Phase III clinical trials are conducted on patients with the same type of cancer to compare the effectiveness of the new treatment with that of the standard treatment being used in the country. In this type of study, half the patients will get the new treatment and half will get the standard treatment. Patients enrolled in a Phase III clinical trial are randomly assigned to be in one of these groups. You cannot select which treatment you want to get.

Participating in a clinical trial is not being a "guinea pig." These studies are designed thoughtfully, building on information we have previously learned about the new treatment. To protect the safety of patients, the U.S. Food and Drug Administration (FDA) strictly regulates and monitors how clinical trials are conducted. The study must undergo internal review at the hospital the doctor is affiliated with and must be approved and monitored by an Institutional Review Board (IRB). In addition, each study has very specific **eligibility criteria** describing who can be treated in the study. A further step to protect people enrolled in clinical trials is that everyone receives a **consent form** describing the purpose of the study, the treatment they will receive, the possible side effects of treatment, the risks and benefits, and the financial costs of treatment. Before receiving any treatment, you must sign this consent form, indicating your understanding of the study and your agreement to participate in it.

Participating in a clinical trial offers you the opportunity to receive new treatments before they are available to other people. You receive care by a leading doctor affiliated with a major cancer center, and you are closely monitored throughout your treatment. You are also able to contribute to progress in medical science. However, it is important to remember that the treatment given in a clinical trial is not yet proven to be more effective than standard treatment you might receive, and there may even be side effects that were not expected. Furthermore, you may have to spend more time receiving treatment, having required diagnostic tests, and seeing the doctor. In addition, there may be more financial costs to you. Some aspects of care may not be covered by your health insurance, and there may be costs of transportation or housing if the treatment is not close to home. There is no right thing to do; the decision as to whether or not to participate in a clinical trial is ultimately yours.

To protect patients, the U.S. Food and Drug Administration strictly regulates and monitors clinical trials.

Eligibility criteria
list of conditions that must be met for someone to enroll in a clinical trial.

Consent form
a written document signed by a patient to indicate that they have been informed about a particular treatment and of the risks and benefits associated with that treatment and agree to receive the treatment; also referred to as "informed consent".

Cancer and Cancer Treatment

17

Although most of the cancer clinical trials are designed to test new treatments for cancer, an increasing number of clinical trials are designed to test new methods of managing symptoms experienced by people with cancer. If you are interested in finding out more about clinical trials, *Taking Part in Clinical Trials: What Cancer Patients Need to Know* is an excellent resource. This is available from the Cancer Information Service of the National Cancer Institute. The following resources provide listings of clinical trials for particular cancers and cancer symptoms:

- National Cancer Institute at *cancer.gov/clinical_trials* or 800-4-CANCER
- National Institutes of Health at *www.clinicaltrials.gov*
- Coalition of National Cancer Cooperative Groups at *cancertrialshelp.org* or 877-520-4457
- Centerwatch, an information services company, provides a listing of clinical trials at *centerwatch.com*

11. What are complementary and alternative treatments?

Complementary and alternative medicine (CAM), also referred to as integrative medicine, includes a wide variety of approaches to improving health and treating disease that are not recognized as standard or conventional by the traditional medical community. When used in addition to conventional methods of treatment, they are referred to as complementary; when used instead of conventional methods of treatment, they are referred to as alternative.

Complementary and alternative therapies may be categorized in many different ways. The National Center for Complementary and Alternative Medicine (NCCAM) divides these into five domains:

1. Alternative medical systems of theory and practice: Many of these are used by different cultures in various parts of the world, for example, Asian, Indian, and Native American Indian practices. **Acupuncture** originated as a part of traditional Chinese medicine. Other examples of alternative medical systems are **homeopathic** and **naturopathic medicine**.

2. Mind–body interventions: These are techniques that aim at helping the mind to enhance various body functions and reduce symptoms. Examples include relaxation, meditation, guided imagery, hypnosis, prayer, and support groups.

3. Biologically based therapies: These include dietary (for example, macrobiotic diet), herbal (for example, saw palmetto), biologic (for example, shark cartilage), and orthomolecular (for example, vitamins) treatments.

4. Manipulative and body-based methods: These are techniques that involve manipulation or movement of the body, such as those used by chiropractors and massage therapists.

5. Energy therapies: These are techniques that manipulate energy fields within or outside of the body, such as therapeutic touch, **Reiki**, or magnets.

The use of complementary and alternative therapies is rapidly increasing. This is in part due to our increasing understanding of them. There is a constantly growing body of scientific knowledge about specific complementary and alternative therapies, how they work, and what effects they have on the body. The U.S. government, to disseminate authoritative information about complementary and alternative therapies and to scientifically study their safety and effectiveness, founded the National Center for Complementary and Alternative Medicine as part of the National Institutes of Health.

Acupuncture
a technique of inserting thin needles into the body at specific locations with the goal of restoring the normal flow of energy in the body; often used to treat pain or other symptoms.

Homeopathic medicine
treatment with extremely small doses of substances that produce symptoms of illness in healthy people when given in larger doses to stimulate the body's own healing responses.

Naturopathic medicine
use of a variety of interventions based on the belief they can enhance the body's natural healing forces.

Reiki
a technique of hands-on touching based on the belief that this touching channels the body's spiritual energy, which leads to spiritual and physical healing.

Cancer and Cancer Treatment

However, the increased use of complementary and alternative therapies also reflects the feeling of desperation many people with cancer have, resulting in a willingness to try anything and everything they feel may help them. Complementary and alternative therapies are not regulated the same way medications and medical devices are. Many treatments and products can be purchased for which there is no evidence of effectiveness. In fact, some of these may even be harmful to you. If you are considering one of these therapies, it is important to get as much accurate information as you can about it. Discuss your thoughts with your doctor and inform him or her of your intentions. Many of these therapies can be used safely with the traditional treatments you are receiving; however, some can interfere with your treatment, cause serious side effects when combined with your treatment, or may by themselves by harmful to you. See Question 18 to learn how to obtain additional information about complementary and alternative therapies.

If you are considering unconventional therapies, get as much accurate information as you can about them.

12. Why do cancer treatments cause side effects?

Despite the most careful considerations of how to safely treat a particular person's cancer, most treatments cause side effects. Surgery to remove the cancer is an important part of the treatment for many types of cancer; however, depending on the type of disease and the extent of surgery performed, there may be changes in how your body looks or functions. Chemotherapy and radiation therapy work primarily by attacking the cancer cell's ability to divide. Because normal cells also need to divide for the body to function normally, they may also be damaged by treatment, causing side effects. Radiation therapy and some types of chemotherapy may also damage particular organs in the body.

Some side effects occur during or shortly after treatment and generally resolve completely after treatment is completed. These are sometimes referred to as acute or early side effects. Examples include drops in blood counts, nausea, vomiting, diarrhea, and mouth sores. Other side effects may not show up for months or years after treatment is completed. These are sometimes referred to as chronic or long-term side effects. Although these are rarer than the acute effects, some are permanent and have the potential to cause significant problems.

Planning treatment for any one person always involves balancing the risks of treatment with the potential benefits. Your doctor will discuss these with you before you begin treatment so that you understand the goals of treatment and the potential side effects you may experience.

Planning treatment always involves balancing the risks with the potential benefits.

13. Is my treatment more likely to work if I get more severe side effects?

Lisa's comment:

Even though I uttered the words "myth" countless times to my own patients, when I experienced minimal side effects from chemotherapy and radiation therapy (at first) I found myself thinking: "I wonder if this is working!" Intellectually, I knew it was, but emotionally . . . . Funny.

A common myth among many people is that when treating cancer, the severity of side effects indicates the effectiveness of treatment. This may even lead people to avoid taking medication to relieve their side effects, thinking it will stop the treatment from working as well. This is not true. Some people who have had successful treatment with long-term cure had minimal

Cancer and Cancer Treatment

side effects from their treatment. Unfortunately, others have a very difficult time with treatment, having severe side effects, even requiring hospitalization, and yet their cancer does not respond to treatment and continues to grow and spread.

The severity of side effects is most commonly linked to the type of treatment you are receiving.

The severity of side effects is most commonly linked to the type of treatment you are receiving. Some treatments are known to cause significant side effects; others are very well tolerated. Your general state of health, your level of activity, and how well you are eating and drinking can also effect how you tolerate treatment. Taking medication to manage any side effects you have will not interfere with the treatment. In fact, it will help you feel better so you can eat and drink well and maintain your usual activities as much as possible.

14. How does my doctor evaluate if my treatment is working? What if my treatment doesn't work?

Throughout your treatment, you will be seeing your doctor regularly so that he or she can evaluate how you are doing. These visits are necessary to see how you are tolerating the treatment, if you are having side effects, and how severe they are. The doctor may order medication to help relieve the side effects and may even make adjustments in your treatment dose or schedule. Another reason for these visits is to see how your cancer is responding to the treatment. If you have had the cancer removed by surgery or destroyed by chemotherapy or radiation therapy, the doctor wants to be sure there is no sign that the cancer has recurred (reappeared). If the cancer could not be removed or destroyed, the doctor wants to be sure it is not progressing (growing) or metastasizing (spreading to other areas). The doctor will review any symptoms you are having and perform a physical examination. Blood tests will be done, and at periodic intervals you will have radiologic studies to see images of the body, such as CT, MRI, or PET. The specific blood tests and radiologic studies depend on the type of cancer you have.

If you are tolerating treatment well and there is no sign that the disease has recurred, progressed, or metastasized, your doctor will continue the treatment. Depending on your situation, the treatment may be planned for a defined period of time (for example, 6 months) or may be given indefinitely. However, if you develop a recurrence or if the tumor progresses or metastasizes while you are on treatment, this indicates that the cancer cells have become resistant to the treatment you are getting. If that happens, your doctor will recommend discontinuing your current treatment and will discuss other options with you. If your energy level is good, if your weight is fairly stable, and if you are able to be up and around most of the day, it is more likely you will have a good response to active treatment, so your doctor will probably recommend a new type of treatment.

It is very distressing to hear that your cancer has recurred after it was removed or that it has grown while you have been on treatment. You may find yourself experiencing again many of the feelings you had when you were first diagnosed: anger, sadness, worry, or even difficulty accepting the reality of what the doctor is telling you. You may feel frightened that you will develop new physical symptoms. You may feel concerned about family and friends. You may be worried about the financial implications for your family. You may feel spiritually distressed. Questions 88–90 have suggestions on how to cope with these emotions and concerns.

Getting accurate information from your doctor will be particularly important as you consider what comes next. Some people find it helpful to have their doctor fully explain the details of their illness and their prognosis. Others prefer not to hear the details and prefer to focus on the plan. Decide what you want to know and communicate this to your family and doctor (see Question 16).

If you have been hoping for cure, hearing that your disease has recurred or grown will challenge the way you have been thinking about your illness.

If you have been hoping for cure, hearing that your disease has recurred or grown will challenge the way you have been thinking about your illness. You may rethink your goals for treatment and reconsider what is most important to you if you cannot be cured. It is important to communicate with your family and with your doctor and nurse about any concerns you have and about the goals you have for yourself. A resource that may be helpful during this time is *When Cancer Recurs: Meeting the Challenge*, published by the National Cancer Institute.

15. What happens after my cancer treatment is completed?

When your treatment is completed, your doctor will schedule regular follow-up visits to be sure you are recovering from treatment, to make sure you have not developed any long-term side effects to treatment, and to evaluate the status of your tumor. Your doctor will review any symptoms you are having, perform a physical examination, draw blood for laboratory analysis, and order radiologic studies to see images of the body, such as CT, MRI, or PET. The specific blood tests and radiologic studies depend on the type of cancer you have. These help the doctor detect if the tumor has grown back (recurrence) or if cells have begun to grow in other parts of the body (metastasis). If all the tests are negative, you have no signs or symptoms of cancer, and there is "no evidence of disease," the doctor may say you are in **remission**. When this continues over a number of years, the doctor may say you are "cured."

Remission
a disappearance of all signs and symptoms of cancer; cancer cells may still be in the body.

Initially, your doctor may want to see you every 2 to 3 months. Over time, the visits will be further apart, going to every 6 months and then to once a year. If you have received combined treatments, ask your doctors to clarify when you should see your surgeon, medical oncologist, and radiation oncologist.

Many people find that the days immediately before their doctor's appointments and the days waiting for the results of diagnostic tests are times of anxiety and worry. Completing treatment for cancer brings other challenges as well. Among these may be adjusting to changes in your body, recovering strength after treatment, resuming your usual activities, returning to work, and explaining your illness to friends and colleagues. In addition, despite the fact that your treatment is over, you may find it difficult at times to balance the hopefulness that the disease will not come back with the knowledge that the future is always uncertain. Each of these challenges presents a new hurdle to overcome. Give yourself time and remember to draw on your usual methods of coping as well as those that are newly learned as you transition into feeling "normal" again (see Question 92).

Completing treatment for cancer brings other challenges as well.

There are three resources that will be particularly helpful to you as you adjust to your life as a cancer survivor:

1. *Facing Forward Series: Life After Cancer Treatment*, published by the National Cancer Institute, covers post-treatment issues such as follow-up medical care, physical and emotional changes, changes in social relationships, and workplace issues.
2. The Cancer Survivors Network of the American Cancer Society, *www.acscsn.org*, offers recorded discussions on particular issues and provides an opportunity to interact with other survivors.
3. The National Coalition for Cancer Survivorship, *www.canceradvocacy.org*, an advocacy organization for cancer survivors, has valuable information, including a Cancer Survival Toolbox.

Despite the fears and uncertainties that lie ahead, some people find that having been diagnosed with cancer provides them the opportunity to think about their lives in new ways. Relationships often become stronger and are enriched by the experience. Sometimes people choose to shift the priorities in their life, ensuring that they are spending their time doing what is most important to them.

PART TWO

Getting Information and Making Decisions

How can I be sure to get the information I want from my doctor?

How can I find a clinical trial that might be appropriate for me?

How can I find out about complementary or alternative therapies?

More . . .

16. How can I be sure to get the information I want from my doctor?

Pete's comment:

Before meeting with my oncologist, I write my questions on an index card. My wife is always with me to ask additional questions and take notes if necessary. By using this approach, I feel much more relaxed and in control. I also find that my oncologist's nurse practitioner is extremely helpful and provides follow up answers to a number of questions.

It is important to feel comfortable with your doctor, to trust his or her medical judgment, and to feel you can communicate with him or her. Doctors will generally try to tell you everything you need to know about your disease and treatment, but they may not tell you everything you want to know. So, first, you must decide what you want to know.

Everyone approaches a diagnosis of cancer differently. Some people want to know every detail about their disease and treatment and prognosis and to be involved in every decision that is made. Others prefer to know only the basics and to have their family or doctor make decisions for them. Of course, many people fall in between. In addition, at different points in time, you may want to know different things. When you are first diagnosed, your concerns will be different from those you may have during treatment or at some point when you are no longer receiving treatment. There may even be some things you never want to know. There is no right way to approach this; however, you should identify what your way is, decide how much you want to know, and communicate this to your family and doctor.

Each time you visit your doctor, decide beforehand what you want to learn at that visit. Talk with members of your family or anyone else you can speak openly with to help focus your thoughts and concerns. Once you have clarified these, write your questions down on a piece of paper. There are no stupid questions, so include everything that concerns you. When you see your doctor, tell him or her at the beginning of the visit that before you leave that day you would like to ask questions. That will help your doctor plan extra time to speak with you. Here are some questions you may want to ask when you first meet with your oncologist:

Each time you visit your doctor, decide beforehand what you want to learn at that visit.

- Is the cancer localized or has it spread to other sites?
- What other diagnostic tests do I need?
- Can this cancer be surgically removed?
- What choices do I have in regard to treatment?
- What treatment do you recommend and why?
- What is the goal of this treatment?
- What are the risks of this treatment?
- How will you know if the treatment is working?
- What are the alternatives to this treatment?
- How will I feel during and after this treatment?
- What side effects will I have from this treatment?
- What do I need to do to care for myself during this treatment?
- Will I be able to work and continue my usual activities during treatment?
- What are reasons I should call your office?

When answering your questions, your doctor may present a lot of information and use terms that are unfamiliar or confusing. As you listen, you may feel anxious or afraid and find it difficult to understand everything that is being said. If there is something you don't understand, ask the doctor to explain it.

If there is something you don't understand, ask the doctor to explain it.

Getting Information and Making Decisions

29

It will help to take notes while the doctor is speaking. Bring a family member or friend with you to be a second set of ears listening to what is said. They can take notes for you while the doctor is speaking and can review the answers with you when you get home. If there is something that is still unclear when you get home, call the office the next day. The nurse who works with your doctor may also be able to answer many of your questions. You are entitled to have your questions answered, so be persistent.

Some patients find they are more comfortable not knowing detailed answers to questions, but they have family members with many questions. Identify one person to be the family spokesperson, coming to office visits and contacting your doctor as needed to ask questions. The family spokesperson can use the same suggestions described above to clarify what everyone wants to know and to be sure to get everyone's questions answered.

17. How can I find a clinical trial that might be appropriate for me?

Clinical trials are research studies designed to test new treatments on humans (see Question 10). Although most clinical trials are designed to test treatments for particular medical problems or types of cancer, some clinical trials test treatments for specific symptoms. If you are interested in participating in a clinical trial, speak with your doctor and see what he or she recommends. If you are looking for a clinical trial to treat your cancer, it may be better to hold off starting treatment until you have investigated the options; you want to discuss if this is appropriate with your doctor. If you are

Clinical trials
research studies to test the effectiveness of new treatments on human beings.

having persistent symptoms or side effects, you may want to first see whether there are other standard treatments available that may help you before enrolling in a clinical trial. If you decide to pursue this possibility, your doctor may be able to help you find clinical trials available for you and can determine if you would be eligible for these.

You can also find out about clinical trials by contacting any of the following organizations:

- National Comprehensive Cancer Center Network (NCCN) at *www.nccn.org*. Select "Network Hospitals" to find a cancer center in your geographic region. Contact them to see if there are any available clinical trials for your cancer or symptom.
- National Cancer Institute at *cancer.gov/clinicaltrials/* or 800-4-CANCER.
- National Institutes of Health at *www.clinicaltrials.gov*. Select "Focused Search" and type in the symptom.
- Coalition of National Cancer Cooperative Groups at *cancertrialshelp.org* or call 877-520-4457.
- Centerwatch, an information services company, provides a listing of clinical trials at *centerwatch.com*.

18. How can I find out about complementary or alternative therapies?

Complementary and alternative medicine (CAM), also referred to as integrative medicine, refers to a wide variety of approaches to improving health and treating disease that are not recognized as standard or conventional by the traditional medical community. When used in addition to conventional methods of treatment, they are referred to as complementary; when used instead of conventional methods of treatment, they are referred to as alternative (see Question 11).

There are several reliable sources of information about complementary and alternative therapies. Because of the rapidly changing state of knowledge about this area of medicine, the Internet will provide the most up-to-date information. The following websites provide general information on complementary and alternative therapies:

- Cancer Information Service of the National Cancer Institute at *cancer.gov/cancerinfo/treatment/cam*
- National Center for Complementary and Alternative Medicine of the National Institutes of Health at *nccam.nih.gov/health/*
- Memorial Sloan-Kettering Cancer Center at *www.mskcc.org/aboutherbs*
- MD Anderson Cancer Center at *www.mdanderson.org/topics/complementary*
- The Richard and Hinda Rosenthal Center for Complementary and Alternative Medicine at Columbia University at *cpmcnet.columbia.edu/dept/rosenthal/CAM_Resources.html*
- American Academy of Medical Acupuncture, *www.medicalacupuncture.org* or 323-937-5514

The following provide information specifically on dietary supplements, including vitamins, minerals, and **botanicals**:

- Office of Dietary Supplements of the National Institutes of Health at *dietary-supplements.info.nih.gov*
- Center for Food Safety and Applied Nutrition of the US Food and Drug Administration at *www.cfsan.fda.gov*
- American Botanical Council at *www.herbalgram.org*

Botanicals

plants or plant parts valued for their medicinal properties; includes herbal products; commonly prepared as a tea, an extract, or a tincture.

The following web site provides scientific biblio-graphic citations related to particular therapies:

- National Library of Medicine at *www.nlm.nih.gov/nccam/camonpubmed.html*

19. How do I decide if I should use one of the complementary or alternative therapies my family or friends are recommending?

Before beginning treatment with any complementary or alternative therapy, obtain as much information as you can about it. Question 18 provides suggestions on how to obtain information. Some specific questions to consider are as follows:

- Do the promises sound too good to be true, for example, promises that are inconsistent with the information you are receiving from your doctor or from other sources of information?
- What is the evidence supporting the claims of effectiveness? Were scientific, rigorously controlled clinical trials conducted? Or, is the evidence only anecdotal, based on the author's personal experience or claims of satisfied customers?
- What are the risks of using this treatment? What is the evidence regarding safety? How are data collected to evaluate safety?
- If a particular person is providing the therapy, what are their qualifications, certifications, or licenses? Some practitioners are now licensed by state medical boards or accredited by professional organizations.
- Is the source of information about the therapy also the seller of the therapy? If that is the case, they may have a vested interest in convincing you to purchase the product.

Two Internet sites provide tips to help in making decisions about using a complementary or alternative therapy:

- National Center for Complementary and Alternative Medicine of the National Institutes of Health at *nccam.nih.gov/health/decisions/index.htm*
- Center for Food Safety and Applied Nutrition of the U.S. Food and Drug Administration at *www.cfsan.fda.gov/~dms/ds-savvy.html*

Before making a definitive decision about the use of any complementary or alternative therapy, discuss your thoughts with your doctor and inform him or her of your intentions.

Before making a definitive decision about the use of any complementary or alternative therapy, discuss your thoughts with your doctor and inform him or her of your intentions. Many of these therapies can be used safely with the traditional treatments you are receiving. However, some can interfere with your treatment, cause serious side effects when combined with your treatment, or may actually be harmful to you.

20. There is so much information on the Internet. How do I evaluate this information to be sure it is complete, accurate, and up-to-date?

Pete's comment:

The sheer amount of information on the Internet can be intimidating and confusing. By concentrating on several credible and reputable sites, I get good background data which increases my knowledge without overwhelming me. I also find that cancer center web sites are a good source of information. If I have questions, I refer to my oncology team for clarification.

The Internet has created the opportunity for you to get instant access to an enormous amount of information without ever leaving your home. However, because there is no control or regulation of the information that is posted on the Internet, a great deal of it may not be accurate.

When viewing a particular site, look for specific elements to help you determine whether the site is a reliable one and likely to have complete, accurate, and up-to-date information. These include the following:

Because there is no regulation of information posted on the Internet, a great deal of it may not be accurate.

- Owner or sponsor of the site: The owner or sponsor of the site pays for it to be maintained. This may be a government agency, a nonprofit organization, a medical center or hospital, a pharmaceutical company, or an individual. The sponsor can influence what content is presented. Consider if the sponsor may benefit by presenting a biased point of view.
- Purpose of the site: The purpose of the site is usually found by clicking "about this site." It should be clearly stated and will help determine whether there is a particular point of view.
- Editorial board: Many sites will have an editorial board that reviews all information posted on the site. Review the list of people on the editorial board and check their credentials and affiliations to be sure they are medically qualified to make these decisions.
- Source of information: The author or authors of the information should be identified. Review their credentials and affiliations to be sure they are truly experts in the field. If the information is obtained from other sources, these should be acknowledged.
- Evidence: References to scientific research findings and published articles that back up the information presented should be included.
- Date information was updated: The site should include a statement indicating the date the informa-

35

tion was last reviewed and updated. Medical information must be current to be useful.

- Privacy: The site may ask for information about you. It should clearly state how the information will be used and how your privacy will be protected.

Before acting on any information you have obtained from the Internet, discuss what you have found and what you are considering with your doctor.

21. I want to have the best quality of life possible. Should I refuse to take any treatment so I won't have side effects?

One of the most difficult aspects of being diagnosed with cancer is living with uncertainty about the future. Coupled with that is the fear of side effects from treatment. These can lead to questioning whether or not it is worthwhile to get treatment. Your decisions about treatment should be based on knowledge, not on fear. Speak with your doctor to get the information you need.

Your decisions about treatment should be based on knowledge, not on fear.

The side effects and the likelihood of long-term control or cure of disease are based on the type of cancer you have, the stage of disease, and the recommended treatment(s). Everyone is different and will respond differently to treatment, so no one can predict precisely what will happen to you. However, your doctor can give you information about what will most likely happen, describing the goals of treatment and the possible risks, and you should consider these when making your decision.

When a cancer is curable, it is often easier to make the decision, because the goal is easy to understand. Many treatments are easily tolerated, with minimal disruption in your usual routines, and many side effects from treatment resolve without any long-term consequences.

Even for those who cannot be cured, there are a number of benefits to obtaining treatment. Many types of cancer can be controlled with treatment for a long period of time. Equally important to consider is that treatment can improve the quality of your life. It can lessen or prevent symptoms of the disease, and it can prevent or delay complications from growth of the cancer.

See Question 16 for specific questions to ask your doctor to ensure you get the information you need to make the decision about undergoing treatment for your cancer.

22. I feel so overwhelmed by all the information I'm getting. How do I make decisions about my treatment?

Pete's comment:

After receiving my lung cancer diagnosis, my wife and I were overwhelmed. We decided to take it one step at a time and move slowly. The first thing we felt was necessary was to get a second opinion at another institution. Our primary concern was being comfortable with the oncologist and his medical team. We also were very aware of the proximity of the potential treatment center and if it was covered by my medical insurance.

After being diagnosed with cancer, one of the most stressful periods of time is when you have to make decisions about your treatment. A number of things can help you sort out the options available to you and select the one that is best for you.

First, be sure you have all the relevant information. Are you clear about your clinical situation and the choices being presented to you? If not, refer to Question 16 for suggestions on how to obtain this information from your doctors.

Second, be sure you have seen all the treating specialists to hear their recommendations directly. An **internist** or surgeon can provide you with direction, but they will not be able to give you detailed information about chemotherapy or radiation therapy. If these treatments are being recommended, schedule appointments with a medical oncologist (who prescribes chemotherapy) and a radiation oncologist (who prescribes radiation therapy). Clarify with each doctor what the goals of treatment are. Also ask about the potential side effects or risks of treatment. See Question 16 for a list of additional questions you may want to ask. This will help you weigh the choices for yourself.

Once you are clear on the options being posed by your doctors, consider if it would be worthwhile to obtain a second opinion, perhaps with a specialist at an academic center or comprehensive cancer center. Doctors who specialize in treating particular types of cancer have more experience with this disease and may have a different perspective about treatment. In addition, they may be able to offer you treatment on a clinical trial.

Have a family member or friend accompany you to all these appointments. They can provide a second set of ears, hearing the information presented, and can take notes for you while the doctors are speaking. When

Internist

a physician who specializes in the diagnosis and medical treatment of adults.

you get home, you will also have someone to review all the information with you to be sure you understand it correctly.

In making your final treatment decision, there are several other factors to consider. Financial issues are important. What are the costs of the various treatment options, including treatment on a clinical trial? Does your health insurance cover treatment by any doctor or only by doctors affiliated with your health insurance plan? Will treatment on a clinical trial be covered? What percentage of the costs will be reimbursed to you and what will be the out-of-pocket expenses? Logistical issues are also important. Where would you have to go for treatment? Will it be easy to get back and forth, or will you have to travel long distances or even relocate to a different city for a period of time? And finally, consider your emotional reactions to the different doctors you have met. Did you feel you could trust the doctor? Did you feel you were given adequate time to have all your questions answered? Did you feel treated respectfully and courteously by the staff in the office? It is important to feel comfortable with the doctor you choose, because he or she will be your partner in the journey that lies ahead.

At the end it comes down to you. Consider everything about your current life situation: how old you are; your general state of health; your responsibilities in regard to family and work; the emotional, physical, and financial costs of treatment; and all that you may possibly gain from treatment. The most difficult part of this process is that there is no "right" decision out there waiting to be found. The right decision is the one that feels right to you.

There is no "right" decision but the one that feels right to you.

23. What is palliative care and how can I get referred to a palliative care program?

Palliative care is a philosophy of care that addresses the medical, physical, emotional, social, and spiritual needs of patients to help them achieve the best possible quality of life. Historically, it was associated with hospice care and was reserved for patients at the end of life who were no longer receiving active treatment for their disease. However, in recent years the focus of palliative care has expanded to include all patients who could benefit from this approach, even those receiving active treatment and with a good prognosis. Many hospitals have established palliative care programs for their patients.

Although oncologists have a great deal of experience in managing pain and other symptoms, for some patients the usual interventions are not effective. In this situation, a referral to a palliative care specialist may be helpful. Palliative care specialists are physicians who are specially trained in techniques to manage pain and other symptoms. If you feel your pain or other symptoms are not well controlled, ask your doctor about seeing a palliative care specialist.

24. What are advance directives? How can I be sure my wishes are known?

Advance directives are legal documents that provide you the opportunity to state what type of medical care you want to receive if you become unable to make decisions or speak for yourself at some time in the future. Although the specific laws and terminology for

Hospice

a program that provides care to patients at the end of their life; can be provided at home or at an in-patient facility.

Advance directives

legal documents in which you indicate who you want to make medical decisions for you and/or what type of medical care you want to receive if you become unable to make decisions or speak for yourself.

advance directives vary from state to state, there are two basic types of advance directives:

- A living will
- A health care proxy

A **living will** is a document in which you can state specific instructions you would like carried out regarding your health care, including measures that would prolong your life. The document could outline which medical interventions you want to have performed and which you want to have withheld for a variety of circumstances.

There are a number of medical interventions you may want to specify in a living will. If you were to lose the ability to eat and drink, what would your wishes be regarding receiving artificial nutrition through a feeding tube or receiving intravenous fluids? If your heart were to stop beating or if you were to stop breathing, what would your wishes be regarding resuscitation: performing cardiopulmonary resuscitation (CPR), putting a tube down your throat and connecting it to a breathing machine, or shocking your heart?

When making these decisions it is helpful to differentiate between the types of problems that could occur. If the problem is treatable and reversible, you may want all medical measures taken to resuscitate you and support you. If the problem results from progressive cancer that can no longer be controlled, you may not want any extraordinary measures taken to resuscitate you or prolong your life. In that situation, some people want to be very explicit about this and request to sign a **"do not resuscitate" (DNR) order** to ensure that none of these measures is taken. Making these decisions is very

Living will
document in which you can state specific instructions regarding your health care, including measures that would prolong your life; may outline which medical interventions you want to have performed and which you want to have withheld for a variety of circumstances.

Do not resuscitate (DNR) order
indication in a patient's medical chart based on the expressed wishes of the patient or their health care proxy that no extraordinary life-extending measures are to be taken if they stop breathing or if their heart stops beating.

41

difficult. You need to think about what you want for yourself, and these documents provide you the opportunity to state this so people can act on your decisions.

There are two limitations to a living will. First, not all states recognize a living will. Second, it is impossible to imagine all the possible circumstances that might occur in regard to your health. There may be decisions to be made that you have not thought to specify in writing. These problems can be avoided by designating a health care proxy.

Health care proxy

a person designated to make health care decisions for you if you are not able to; also called a health care surrogate, a medical proxy, or a medical power of attorney.

A **health care proxy**, also called a health care surrogate, a medical proxy, or a medical power of attorney, authorizes a designated person to make health care decisions for you if you are not able to. They can decide which medical interventions should be performed and which should be withheld. Although the terminology varies from state to state, all states recognize a health care proxy.

When selecting a health care proxy, be sure to choose someone you trust and someone who will make decisions based on what you want for yourself, not on what they want for you or on what they would want for themselves if they were in your position. You can choose a family member or a friend as your health care proxy. Talk with the person about what you want for yourself in a variety of circumstances. Talk about the issues described above, in regard to resuscitation and life-prolonging measures like artificial nutrition and intravenous fluid. Be as specific as you are able to be. Then confirm with the person that he or she will honor your wishes and are willing to speak for you. You can change your health care proxy, and you can change your decisions about what you want done, at any time.

Let your family and friends know whom you have selected as your health care proxy so that if the need arises for them to act on this, everyone can support this person in making the decisions that may have to be made. If you have completed a living will, share this with them as well. Inform all of your doctors and everyone else in the medical team caring for you of your wishes and provide them with copies of any advance directive documents you have signed.

Having a discussion about what you would want if you were unable to make decisions for yourself is difficult for most people. Sometimes the person who is ill wants to bring it up but is afraid the family will be distressed by the conversation. Sometimes the family wants to bring it up but is afraid of harming the person by discussing these painful issues. It is always better to talk about these things when you are feeling fairly well and there is no imminent crisis looming overhead. This way you will be able to calmly think about what you want and clearly talk about this with each other.

There are several ways you can initiate the discussion. You could say something like "I want to be sure that if I were to become sicker you would know what I want done." A family member could initiate the discussion by saying something like "If you were to become sicker and couldn't tell me what kind of care you wanted, I would not know what to do. Can we talk about this?" Some people find that their family does not agree with the decisions they have made. This can make a difficult discussion even more difficult. In a situation like this, it is particularly helpful to have an advance directive to ensure your wishes will be honored.

You can obtain state-specific advance directive documents from your lawyer, your doctor, or your local hospital. The Partnership for Caring, a nonprofit organization whose mission is to improve how people die, also provides state-specific documents. In addition, they provide information on end-of-life issues and offer a national crisis and information hotline dealing with these issues. They can be contacted at *www.partnershipforcaring.org/ Advance/index.html* or 800-989-9455.

PART THREE

Comfort, Activity, and Sleep

Will I have pain? What are the options
available to treat my pain?

What can I do about the side effects
I get from my pain medication?

I feel tired much of the time.
What can I do to increase my energy?

I have difficulty sleeping at night.
What can I do to sleep better and feel more rested?

More . . .

COPING WITH PAIN

25. Will I have pain? What are the options available to treat my pain?

Pete's comment:

When I was first diagnosed, I had peripheral pain which would flare up in my back throughout the day. I was put on Tylenol #3 (acetaminophen with codeine) to help manage it. This worked well and after several sessions of chemotherapy, the pain subsided and I was able to cut back on the medication. Eventually, the pain disappeared completely.

Pain has long been considered to be an unavoidable consequence of having cancer. However, with the development of new pain medications and with increasing understanding of how to use these more effectively, cancer pain can be well controlled in almost all people.

Not everyone with cancer develops pain.

Not everyone with cancer develops pain. If a tumor grows or spreads, it may press on or invade surrounding organs or nerves. Depending on the location of the tumor, this may cause pain. In addition, procedures used to diagnose or treat cancer may cause pain, for example, having a biopsy to take a sample of tissue to diagnose the type of cancer or having surgery to remove all or part of the tumor.

Pain may be experienced in many different ways, for example, as discomfort, aching, a gnawing feeling, a sharp stabbing sensation, or cramping. It may be mild and intermittent or severe and continuous.

Many people are concerned about taking pain medication. Some people feel it is important to withstand the pain as a sign of strength. Some people feel it is a part of having cancer that they have to accept. Some people are afraid of "masking" a problem and that if they treat the pain their doctor will not be able to follow their response to treatment. There is no benefit at all in having pain. Regardless of how mild the pain is, having chronic pain can be very disabling. It affects your energy level, your appetite, your ability to sleep, your desire to be with friends and family, and your mood. Tell your doctor or nurse about any discomfort you have, no matter how mild it is. Try to describe it accurately so they can decide on the best treatment for you and monitor how effectively that treatment is working. When describing your discomfort, try to tell them about the following things:

There is no benefit at all in having pain.

- Where you feel the pain.
- How severe the pain is. Many doctors and nurses will ask you to rate the severity, for example, using a scale of 0 to 10, with 0 being no pain at all and 10 being the worst pain you can imagine.
- What the pain feels like (for example, sharp, achy, gnawing).
- Whether you have the pain all the time or only at certain times.
- What makes it worse and what makes it better.
- How it affects your ability to sleep, your appetite, your activity, your desire to be with friends and family, and your mood.

Medications for treating pain are called **analgesics**. There are many different analgesics available, and these are often prescribed in a step-wise approach, starting with a mild analgesic and progressing to a stronger one as needed until your pain is controlled. First-line over-

Analgesics
medications to treat pain.

Comfort, Activity, and Sleep

47

the-counter analgesics include acetaminophen, aspirin, and nonsteroidal antiinflammatory drugs (for example, ibuprofen, naproxen). COX-2 inhibitors are a new category of nonsteroidal antiinflammatory medications that are less irritating to the stomach but require a prescription (for example, celecoxib, rofecoxib, valdecoxib). If these medications are not effective, your doctor will prescribe an opioid or narcotic analgesic (for example, morphine, oxycodone, hydromorphone, fentanyl). There are other medications that are effective in relieving pain when used in combination with analgesics. These include certain antidepressant, anticonvulsant, antiinflammatory, and steroid medications.

Pain medications come in many forms: tablets, liquids to swallow, liquids that are absorbed under the tongue, skin patches, and rectal suppositories. There are also solutions that can be given intravenously (into the vein) via a portable pump. The pump is often set to deliver a steady dose of medication into the bloodstream with extra doses that you can deliver as needed. The pump is set up to allow "patient-controlled" medication administration with a limit to prevent overdose.

Pain medication for chronic pain works most effectively when it is given on a regular schedule "around the clock." This keeps a steady level of pain medication in your bloodstream, to prevent you from experiencing pain. New long-acting medications are very helpful because they last for many hours, or even days. To keep your pain controlled with these, you do not need to take medication as frequently as with the immediate-release (short-acting) forms of the medication. However, even with long-acting medication, most people also require an immediate-release pain medication for "break-through" pain. Break-through pain is pain or discomfort that you experience during the day or night despite taking the long-acting medication around the clock. When using the immediate-release pain medication, take it as frequently as you need to. If you wait too long between doses and the pain becomes severe, the medication will not work as quickly or as effectively. If you find you need the immediate-release pain medication very frequently during the day or that it is not effective, ask your doctor about increasing the dose of the long-acting medication.

Some people are concerned about taking pain medication because they are afraid that if they take it for milder pain, it won't work when they might need it later for severe pain. Many pain medications, particularly narcotics, have no maximal dose that can be given. The dose can be increased indefinitely over time, so you can be sure to get good pain relief if you need it at some point in the future, no matter how severe your pain may be.

There are many different types of pain medication, and what works for one person may not work as well for another. It may take some time to find the right medication and the right dose and schedule to keep you without pain. Be persistent in working with your doctor and nurse until you find a regimen that works for you. If you do not feel satisfied with the degree of relief you are getting, ask them about a referral to a pain specialist. You can also find a pain specialist by calling the Cancer Information Service of the National Cancer Institute or the American Cancer Society.

It may take time to find the medication, dose, and schedule that will keep you without pain.

Comfort, Activity, and Sleep

> **There are several reasons to call your doctor about pain:**
> - You are not getting adequate pain relief from your medicine.
> - On a scale of 0 to 10, with 0 being no pain and 10 being the worst pain you can imagine, your pain is at a level of 5 or higher most of the time.
> - You are not able to sleep because of pain.
> - You are not taking the full dose of pain medicine because of the side effects of the medicine.

26. What can I do about the side effects I get from my pain medication?

Pete's comment:

My pain medication, like most, had a side effect of constipation. This was managed by a combination of Colace and Senokot. I also included prunes in my diet and drank plenty of fluids. After several weeks, constipation was no longer a problem and I was able to eliminate the medication.

Some people are concerned about taking pain medication because of the side effects. Common side effects from pain medication include sleepiness, nausea, and constipation. Sleepiness generally passes after a few days. However, if this persists ask your doctor or nurse about adjusting the dose or adding another medication to counteract the sleepiness. Nausea also commonly passes after a few days on pain medication. If you have persistent nausea, ask your doctor about trying a different pain medication or about taking medication to relieve the nausea. Unfortunately, constipation from pain medications does not pass. Taking a combination of a stool softener (for example, docusate) and a laxative (for example, senna, bisacodyl, lactulose, polyethylene glycol) on a regular basis can help. Ask your doctor or nurse about which medications you should take, what dose, and how often you should take these. Increasing the amount of liquid you drink during the day will also help reduce the likelihood of constipation. If you become dizzy or confused from the pain medication, tell your doctor or nurse. Switching the dose or type of medication will usually resolve these problems.

27. I am afraid of taking my pain medication because I don't want to get addicted. What should I do?

Some people are concerned about taking pain medication because they are afraid of becoming addicted. Pain medication does not cause **addiction**; however, when taken on a regular basis it does cause tolerance. This is when your body physically adjusts to the level of medication in your bloodstream. If you stop the medication suddenly, you can develop withdrawal symptoms. Tapering down the dose of medication gradually if you no longer need it, rather than stopping it suddenly, can prevent this. Your doctor or nurse will review with you exactly how to do this. Tolerance to the medication is not addiction, which is a desire or craving for the medication to feel high rather than to have your pain relieved. Research studies show that it is extremely rare for patients with cancer to develop addiction from pain medication.

Addiction
an uncontrollable psychological craving for a substance such as a drug or alcohol.

Pain medication does not cause addiction.

28. Are there other treatments for pain that do not rely on taking medication?

For some types of pain, surgery may be helpful by removing all or part of the tumor that is causing the pain. However, this is not an option for many people, and other treatments are then considered.

Radiation therapy is effective in treating some types of cancer pain. With external beam radiation therapy, a beam of energy is directed from a treatment machine at precise angles toward a defined target in your body. It can reduce pain by shrinking a tumor that is pressing on or invading surrounding organs or nerves. If you do not feel your pain is controlled adequately with the medication you are taking, ask your doctor if radiation therapy would be helpful in treating the type of pain you have. However, if your cancer has spread widely through your body, external beam radiation is unlikely to be effective for you.

For people who have bone metastasis (spread of the primary tumor to the bone) in multiple areas of the body, treatment with a radioactive isotope may be helpful. Strontium-89 is injected into the blood, travels through the body, and collects in the bone where the tumors have spread. It emits radiation to those areas to shrink the tumors, thus reducing the pain they cause.

Nerve block

a procedure in which alcohol or a local anesthetic is injected into or around a nerve to treat pain.

If pain is caused by pressure on a nerve, a procedure called a **nerve block** can sometimes be performed. This involves injecting a local anesthetic or alcohol into or around the nerve near the point where the tumor is pressing. This blocks the transmission of messages from the nerve up to the brain, so you will no longer be aware of the pressure. This may also be done surgically; the nerves are cut to relieve the pain. If you do not feel your pain is controlled adequately with the medication you are taking, ask your doctor if this would be helpful for you.

There are a variety of other strategies that may be helpful in treating pain, either alone or in combination with your pain medication. These include distraction, relaxation, imagery, prayer, meditation, and acupuncture. There are specialists who can perform these or train you in how to use these techniques to control your pain. If you are interested in any of these, ask your doctor or nurse for a referral or contact the National Center for Complementary and Alternative Medicine.

For more information on how to manage pain, the National Cancer Institute has a booklet entitled *Pain Control: A Guide for People with Cancer and Their Families*. This is available on the Internet at *cancer.gov/cancerinfo/paincontrol* or can be ordered over the phone by calling the Cancer Information Service at 800-4-CANCER. Another resource to learn more about pain and how to manage it is the Oncology Nursing Society; information is available on the Internet at *www.cancersymptoms.org/symptoms/pain/*.

29. What can I do for flu-like symptoms?

Flu-like symptoms may be caused by cancer, treatment for cancer, or infections. Flu-like symptoms most commonly include fever, chills, muscle aches (**myalgias**), and fatigue. There may also be decreased appetite, headache, nausea, vomiting, or diarrhea.

Myalgias
aches and pains in the muscles.

If you experience these symptoms, call your doctor or nurse. Unless this is a known chronic problem, you should always report fever of 100.5°F with or without chills to your doctor's office immediately. If these symptoms are new, your doctor will need to make sure you don't have an infection. He or she will ask you questions, perform a physical examination, take blood samples, and perhaps perform other tests. If you have an infection, he or she will prescribe treatment for you.

When flu-like symptoms are caused by your cancer, this is commonly referred to as "tumor fever." Many people with tumor fever will experience symptoms on a daily basis and usually at the same time (or times) each day. Very often treatment of the cancer resulting in remission or cure will eliminate tumor fever.

Flu-like symptoms can also be caused by certain treatments for cancer. If these symptoms are likely to occur from your treatment or from other medicines, your doctor or nurse will tell you. The reaction can occur while you are receiving the medication, within a few hours, or even several days after the treatment. Flu-like symptoms can be caused by

- Chemotherapy, such as gemcitabine, dacarbazine, and bleomycin;
- Biologic therapy (therapy that boosts your immune system to fight the cancer), such as interferon or interleukin, and monoclonal antibodies, such as rituximab and trastuzumab;
- Medicines to strengthen bone, such as pamidronate and zoledronic acid.

If you are likely to experience these symptoms while you are receiving the medication, the doctor or nurse will give you premedication (before the treatment) to prevent the reaction. Premedication can include acetaminophen, diphenhydramine, nonsteroidal antiinflammatory medication (ibuprofen, naproxen), or even meperidine or morphine.

If you experience flu-like symptoms at home, regardless of the reason, the following measures may help:

- Your doctor may prescribe acetaminophon or nonsteroidal antiinflammatory medicines (for example, naproxen) for you to take around-the-clock (on a regular basis).
- Drink plenty of fluids to prevent dehydration from fever.
- Take cool to tepid sponge baths to help keep your fever down.
- Take regular uninterrupted rest periods if you are tired.
- Ask your doctor to prescribe medicine for nausea, vomiting, and diarrhea if you develop these (see Questions 55 to 57 for more information)

30. What can I do to treat itching?

Itching is a sensation that makes people feel the urge to scratch. The medical term for this is **pruritus**. Itching can occur on one area of the body (localized) or it can affect the entire body (generalized). It may be accompanied by a rash or other skin changes. In patients with cancer, itching can have many different causes:

Pruritus
itching.

- Some cancers may be associated with itching, including leukemia, lymphoma, and cancers of the stomach, lung, or breast.
- Some chemotherapy medicines may cause itching, for example, doxorubicin and gefitinib.
- Radiation therapy may cause skin changes, including itching.
- Some medicines can cause itching, including pain medicine (narcotic analgesics like morphine) and antibiotics.
- An allergic reaction to medicine can cause itching.
- Other diseases, such as liver disease (**jaundice**) and kidney failure, may be associated with itching.
- Other causes are dry skin, insect bites, and changes in soap or laundry detergent.

Jaundice
yellowing of the skin and the whites of the eyes resulting from buildup of bilirubin in the tissues; can occur if the bile ducts are blocked or if the liver is not functioning; accompanied by darkening of the urine and lightening of the color of the stools.

Constant scratching can cause more irritation to the skin and, in some people, may cause a break in the skin that can cause additional discomfort and even infection. Itching can interfere with sleep and overall quality of life. If you have itching, a rash, redness, or breakdown of your skin, contact your doctor or nurse before applying anything to your skin. They will ask you many questions and will inspect your skin. They may also want to take a blood sample. Be prepared to give them the following information:

Contact your doctor or nurse before applying anything to your skin to soothe irritation.

• The area that is affected, when it started, and what makes it better or worse.
• Medicines that you are taking, including prescription and over-the-counter medicine. Be sure to tell them if there are any new medicines.
• Changes in your skin, such as rash, hives, or dryness, and changes in the color of your skin, such as redness or yellow skin (jaundice)

If the cancer is causing the itching, treatment resulting in remission or cure will often stop the itching. If the itching is caused by a medicine, they may stop the medicine or switch to another one that will not cause itching. If you have itchiness or a skin reaction from radiation treatments, you should speak to your nurse about specific skin recommendations for people taking radiation therapy.

There are many different treatments for itching. General measures that almost anyone can try are as follows:

• Bathe or shower using tepid water and a superfatted unscented soap (for example, Dove). Aveeno oatmeal baths may be soothing.
• Use emollient lotions such as Curel or Lubriderm.
• Keep fingernails trimmed.
• Keep air humidified.

- Drink plenty of fluids.
- Wear loose-fitting cotton clothing; use cotton sheets.
- Apply cool compresses for localized itching
- Use distraction measures, relaxation techniques, or guided visual imagery.

Treatments that may be prescribed by your doctor or nurse include

- Steroid creams, either by prescription or over the counter;
- Topical or oral antihistamines (for example, diphen-hydramine);
- Sedatives for those who are unable to sleep;
- Referral to a dermatologist for a consultation.

Lisa's comment:

Pruritis associated with the radiation field drove me crazy. Even though I used all recommended creams (Biafine, Bactroban Ointment, Betamethasone Dipropionate Ointment), I still found myself scratching absentmindedly. I felt that I needed to put myself in mittens, in addition to keeping my fingernails short, in order to not cause significant skin breakdown.

ACTIVITY AND SLEEP

31. I feel tired much of the time. What can I do to increase my energy?

Lisa's comment:

I am a single professional woman. I have elderly parents who live across town, a brother who lives 15 miles away, and numerous friends who live both near and far. I am an independent individual. I insisted on getting myself to and from my treatments (chemotherapy) via mass transporta-

tion, alone—I live about 30 miles from the Cancer Center. My fatigue was significant, but generally occurred a few days after treatment. My parents and friends wanted to drive me to my treatments, but I wouldn't allow them. My mother, therefore, took on the added chore of doing my laundry and food shopping every week. My parents' help significantly contributed to my increased energy levels. It allowed me to save my energy for long workdays.

Fatigue is a common problem for people with cancer. It may be experienced as feeling tired, weak, or weary; lacking energy; being unable to concentrate; or feeling irritable or depressed. Many things may cause fatigue. These include the disease itself, the treatment you are receiving, the side effects of certain medications (for example, medications to treat pain or nausea), **anemia** (low red blood cell count), a decrease in the amount of food you eat, a decrease in the amount of liquids you drink, difficulty sleeping, emotional distress, and chronic pain. However, many people with cancer develop fatigue without any clear single cause.

Anemia

a condition in which the number of red blood cells is below normal.

Sleeping extra hours at night, by going to bed earlier or staying in bed a bit later in the morning, will help improve your energy. Resting during the day is also important, napping for short periods or just laying down and relaxing. Plan these rest periods for times when you know you will be more likely to feel tired. For some people, even bathing, dressing, or eating may cause you to feel tired, and it will help to plan time for a short rest after these activities. However, at the same time, you want to push yourself to be as active as you are able to. Lying in bed all day will generally make you weaker. In fact, there is evidence that exercising will actually increase your energy level as long as you don't push yourself to the point of exhaustion. If you are currently exercising on a regular basis, try to maintain this, adjusting the intensity and frequency of your exercise regimen based on how you feel. If you are not currently exercising, take a daily walk. Start with 5 to 15 minutes a day. Adjust the distance and pace based on how you feel. The key thing is finding a balance between rest and activity.

Find a balance between rest and activity.

One cause of fatigue is anemia (low red blood cell count). This may be treated with a medication called epoetin (Procrit, Epogen) or darbepoetin (Aranesp). This medication stimulates your bone marrow to make more red blood cells, raising your blood cell count and increasing your energy. It is given by injection under the skin using a very small thin needle. It comes in different doses and is most commonly given once a week. You may be instructed to take an iron supplement by mouth while getting these injections. If you are anemic and feel fatigued, ask your doctor if this medication could help you.

If there are other specific problems you have that you think may be contributing to your fatigue, speak with your doctor or nurse about these. Ask them about taking a sleeping medication if you are having difficulty sleeping at night. Ask them about how to better manage your pain if you are not comfortable. Ask about how you can better cope with your emotional distress. Ask them for advice on how to increase your food and fluid intake if you feel you are not eating and drinking enough. Unfortunately, fatigue cannot always be effectively treated. It is often necessary to adjust your activity to accommodate to the changes in your energy level.

It is important to conserve your energy for those things that are most important to you. You need to think about all the things you do during the day: work, shopping, cooking, cleaning, household chores, errands, taking care of children or dependent relatives, being with family and friends, and recreational or leisure activities. Which of these activities are most important to you? Which give you the most pleasure? Which make you feel good about yourself? These are the things you want to save your energy for. You will probably notice that your energy is greater at certain times of the day. Plan these activities for those times. For the other things that must get done, ask family and friends for help. People often want to be helpful, but don't know how. Tell them specifically what you need help with; they will probably be grateful for the direction. See Question 96 for suggestions on how family and friends can help. And finally, let go of the things you don't need to do and don't want to do.

To learn more about fatigue and how to manage it, go to the Internet site sponsored by the Oncology Nursing Society at *www.cancersymptoms.org/symptoms/fatigue/* and the National Comprehensive Cancer Network at *www.nccn.org* and view the treatment guidelines for patients, selecting fatigue.

32. I have difficulty sleeping at night. What can I do to sleep better and feel more rested?

Difficulty sleeping is a common problem for many people—either difficulty falling asleep in the evening or difficulty staying asleep throughout the night. Aside from the distress of lying awake in bed for many hours, not getting enough sleep may cause you to feel irritable and tired throughout the day and to have difficulty concentrating.

Try to determine if there is a concrete reason that you are having difficulty sleeping. Are you physically uncomfortable or in pain? Are you having other symptoms, like nausea, vomiting, diarrhea, constipation, itching, mouth sores, or anything else that is making it difficult to sleep? Take medication as prescribed to treat these problems and allow you to get a restful night's sleep. If you are taking medication and it is not effective, tell your doctor or nurse.

Are you feeling anxious and worried during the night? Are your thoughts racing and keeping you awake at night? Speak with someone you trust and feel supported by about your thoughts and feelings; this may provide a significant amount of relief. See Questions 88 to 89 which discuss emotional reactions that people with cancer may experience and suggest ways of feeling more in control. For some people, medication for anxiety may be helpful.

Do you feel generally restless at night, unable to relax and sleep? A variety of techniques may be helpful:

- Establish a regular schedule each day of the times you go to bed at night and awaken in the morning.
- Even if you do not sleep well at night, try not to sleep excessively during the day. This will disrupt your body's normal cycle. If you are very tired, take a short nap during the day, but for only about an hour.
- Avoid being in bed at any time except when you are going to sleep. When resting during the day, lay in another room, on a couch or chair. Use your bed only for sleep at night.
- Avoid drinking caffeine or stimulants after dinner.

Try to determine if there is a concrete reason that you are having difficulty sleeping.

Comfort, Activity, and Sleep

For some people, these techniques will not be helpful. If you continue to have difficulty with sleep, ask your doctor to prescribe a sleeping medication. Getting a restful sleep at night is important to feeling energized and capable during the day.

33. I have seen a commercial about medicine to treat fatigue from cancer treatment. What is this and should I be getting it?

One cause of fatigue is anemia, a low red blood cell count. Red blood cells are produced in the bone marrow and released into the bloodstream where they carry oxygen from the lungs to all the tissues of the body. The cells use oxygen to create energy. When the red blood cell count is low, there is less oxygen available to the cells, resulting in fatigue.

The number of cells in the blood can be measured by testing a blood sample for a complete blood count (CBC). The number of red cells is also reflected in measurements called **hematocrit** (the percentage of red cells in the blood) and **hemoglobin** (the amount of the molecule in the red cells that carries the oxygen). The normal ranges for these tests vary from laboratory to laboratory, but in general normal values are as follows:

Hematocrit

the proportion of blood which is red blood cells; used as a measure of the amount of red blood cells.

Hemoglobin

substance in red blood cells that binds to oxygen and carries it to the tissues of the body; used as a measure of the amount of red blood cells.

- Hemoglobin   12–18 grams per deciliter (g/dl)
- Hematocrit   36–54%

There are many causes of fatigue (see Question 30), but if it is caused by anemia and the hemoglobin is less than 10 g/dl, treatment with a medication called epoetin (Procrit, Epogen) or darbepoetin (Aranesp) may be helpful. This medication stimulates your bone marrow to make more red blood cells, raising your blood cell count and increasing your energy. It is given by injection under the skin using a very small thin needle. It comes in different doses and is most commonly given once a week. You may be instructed to take an iron supplement by mouth while getting these injections. If you are anemic and feel fatigued, ask your doctor if this medication could help you.

Medications that stimulate red blood cell production raise your blood cell count and increase your energy.

34. Can I exercise?

Pete's comment:

Exercise has been an integral part of my life for the last twenty years and I was concerned that my cancer treatment might cause me to cut back. I was encouraged by my oncology team to ease back into an exercise regimen as quickly as possible. I started with chair aerobics and one-on-one personal training with a clinical nurse specialist. I was eventually able to get back to a full workout routine at my gym which has given me both a mental and physical lift.

The benefits of exercise are well known. The American Cancer Society and other organizations recommend exercise for health promotion and prevention of many diseases (for example, heart disease, high blood pressure, cancer). Many studies have shown that exercise may play a role in the prevention of breast, prostate, and colon cancers.

Some people believe that they should "conserve their energy" during the diagnosis, treatment, and recovery phases of cancer. Having a diagnosis of cancer does not mean you have to stop exercising. Studies have shown

Comfort, Activity, and Sleep

*People with
cancer benefit
in multiple
ways from
exercise.*

that people with cancer benefit in multiple ways from exercise, including

- Reduced feelings of anxiety, stress, and depression;
- Decreased treatment-related side effects (nausea, constipation, and fatigue);
- Improved appetite and sleep;
- Improved bone strength and muscular flexibility;
- Improved quality of life and feelings of general well-being.

*If exercise was
a part of your
routine before
cancer diag-
nosis, continue
it during di-
agnosis and
treatment.*

Before exercising, you should check with your doctor or nurse to see whether you should avoid some types of exercise. For most people, there are no limitations regarding exercise. If exercise was a part of your routine before cancer diagnosis, the same routine can usually be continued during diagnosis and treatment. After some types of surgery (breast surgery, lung surgery) your doctor or nurse will recommend specific exercises. Exercise should not cause pain or discomfort. You should participate in activities that are enjoyable.

If you have been in bed for a prolonged period or have not exercised in a long time, performing everyday activities yourself is a good way to get started. Adding exercise to your daily routine can be as simple as taking a walk outside to get the paper or mail, doing light housekeeping, or shopping for food. In general, it is important to start slowly and increase your exercise level gradually.

Others may enjoy yoga or other structured exercise classes offered at fitness centers. Additionally, exercise and yoga videotapes are available at public libraries for those who want to work out at home. Some people participate in aerobic exercise and weight training activities. Studies have shown that structured exercise programs helped cancer patients improve endurance, strength, flexibility, and return to everyday activity faster than those who did not exercise.

There may be specific exercise groups in your area for cancer survivors or those who are actively undergoing cancer treatment. Your local chapter of the American Cancer Society may be able to direct you to a program. Additionally, some hospitals and universities have wellness programs (including nutrition and exercise) for people with cancer. Local fitness centers (for example, the YMCA) may also provide classes for those undergoing cancer treatments. Members of your health care team will be able to provide you with information regarding local resources.

Comfort, Activity, and Sleep

PART FOUR

Blood Counts and Skin Problems

I have heard that chemotherapy may
cause drops in my blood counts.
What does this mean?

I have heard that radiation therapy
causes a skin reaction.
Is this true? How should I care for
my skin during radiation therapy?

I have heard that chemotherapy
may cause me to lose my hair.
Can I prevent this? What can I do to feel
good about my appearance if I lose my hair?

More . . .

Blood Counts and Your Immune System

35. I have heard that chemotherapy may cause drops in my blood counts. What does this mean?

Blood cells are produced in the bone marrow and released into the bloodstream where they are able to protect the body in a variety of ways. **White cells** are part of the immune system and fight off infection. **Platelets** stop bleeding if you are cut or injured by clumping together to plug up damaged blood vessels. **Red cells** carry oxygen from the lungs to all the tissues of the body, where the cells use it to create energy. The number of cells in the blood can be measured by testing a blood sample for a complete blood count (CBC). The number of red cells is also reflected in measurements called hematocrit (the percentage of red cells in the blood) and hemoglobin (the amount of the molecule in the red cells which carries the oxygen). The normal ranges for a CBC vary from laboratory to laboratory, but in general normal values are as follows:

- White blood cells 4–10,000 cells per cubic millimeter (cells/mm³)
- Platelets 150,000–500,000 cells/mm³
- Hemoglobin 12–18 g/dl
- Hematocrit 36–54%

Once the blood cells are released into the bloodstream, they only live for a short time: as short as 24 hours for some types of white cells, about 10 days for platelets, and about 3 months for red cells. The body depends on the rapidly dividing cells in the bone marrow to continuously replace these cells as they die.

White blood cells

cells in the blood that fight off infection and other types of disease; also called leukocytes; there are many different types of white blood cells that include neutrophils and lymphocytes.

Platelets

blood cells that help prevent bleeding by causing clots to form when a blood vessel is cut; also called thrombocytes.

Red blood cells

cells in the blood that contain hemoglobin that carries oxygen from the lungs to all the tissues in the body; also called erythrocytes.

Chemotherapy destroys tumor cells by preventing them from dividing. Normal cells that divide rapidly are very sensitive to the effects of chemotherapy. The cells in the bone marrow lose the ability to form new blood cells so fewer cells are released into the bloodstream. After chemotherapy is given, the blood counts drop, generally 7 to 14 days after treatment. The white cells and platelets are particularly sensitive, because they only live a short period of time. The body can adjust to slight decreases in the number of blood cells without any problem; however, your doctor will order a CBC before you get each cycle of chemotherapy to be sure that your counts are not too low. If your white cell or platelet counts are too low, your doctor may decide to hold your treatment for a week to give the bone marrow a chance to make new blood cells. See Questions 35 to 37 for other measures that may be taken if your blood counts are low.

Radiation therapy may also cause a drop in your blood cell counts. This occurs if the radiation therapy is directed to an area in which a large amount of active bone marrow will be exposed, for example, the pelvis, the ribs, or the spinal column. If there is a chance that your blood cell counts will drop during treatment, your doctor will order a CBC every week or two during your treatment.

36. What do I do if my white blood cell count is low?

If your white blood cell (WBC) count drops, your doctor will want to know which particular types of white blood cells are low. He or she will order a CBC that lists the different types of white blood cells found and the number of each. **Neutrophils** make up about

Neutrophils
A type of white blood cell that fights infection and other diseases.

69

45–75% of your white blood cells; they are an important defense against bacterial infections, and if they are low you have an increased risk of developing an infection. Throughout your treatment, there are things you can do to prevent infection:

- Wash your hands frequently with soap and water, especially before eating and after going to the bathroom.
- Bathe daily with soap and water, and brush your teeth after each meal.
- Avoid people with colds or flu.
- Avoid sharing food utensils, drinking glasses, or toothbrushes.
- Avoid handling feces or urine of pets, especially in cat litter or birdcage droppings.
- Check with your doctor or nurse before having any dental work or immunizations.

Neutropenia

A decrease in the number of neutrophils, the type of white blood cell that fights infection and other diseases.

Your doctor or nurse may advise you to take extra precautions to prevent infection.

If your WBC count drops very low, particularly your neutrophils, this is referred to as **neutropenia**. Your doctor or nurse may advise you to take extra precautions to prevent infection. In addition, your doctor may prescribe a medication called filgrastim (Neupogen) or pegfilgrastim (Neulasta) that can stimulate the bone marrow to make new white cells quickly. It is injected under your skin with a small thin needle. You or a family member may be taught to give the injection at home.

Despite doing all the right things, you may still develop an infection. If you have any implanted catheters or tubes (such as a port, a urinary stent, or a biliary stent) you have a higher than normal risk of developing an infection. You will not feel that your WBC count is low, so call your doctor or nurse if you develop any signs or symptoms of infection. You will most likely need to be examined and have tests taken to determine whether you require treatment with antibiotics.

> **Reasons to call the doctor include**
> - **Fever of 100.5°F or 38°C;**
> - **Shaking chills;**
> - **Sore throat or cough;**
> - **Frequency or burning when you urinate;**
> - **Swelling, redness, or pain anywhere on your skin;**
> - **Vomiting or diarrhea unrelated to your chemotherapy.**

To learn more about neutropenia and how to manage it, go to the Internet site sponsored by the Oncology Nursing Society at *www.cancersymptoms.org/symptoms/ neutropenia/.*

37. What do I do if my platelet count is low?

If your platelet count drops, there is an increased risk of bleeding. Throughout your treatment, unless prescribed by your doctor, avoid aspirin, products that contain aspirin, and nonsteroidal antiinflammatory drugs (NSAIDs), such as ibuprofen, because these may all interfere with platelet functioning. If the platelet count drops very low, your doctor or nurse may advise you to take extra precautions to prevent bleeding, such as using only an electric razor and avoiding activities in which you could be injured.

If your platelet count drops, there is an increased risk of bleeding.

You will not feel that your platelet count is low, so call your doctor or nurse if you develop any signs or symptoms of bleeding.

> **Reasons to call the doctor include**
> - **Easy bruising;**
> - **Bleeding gums or nose bleeds;**
> - **Blood in the urine or stool;**
> - **Black stools.**

38. What do I do if my red blood cell count is low?

If the red blood cell (RBC) count drops, you will feel fatigued. Fatigue can be experienced in many different ways: a lack of energy; feeling tired, weak, or weary; feeling irritable or depressed; or having difficulty concentrating. You may even feel light-headed or short of breath. For suggestions on how to conserve energy and manage fatigue, see Question 30.

If the RBC count falls very low, your doctor may recommend a medication called epoetin (Procrit, Epogen) or darbepoetin (Aranesp) that stimulates the bone marrow to make more red blood cells. It is given by injection under the skin using a very small thin needle. It comes in different doses and can be given either three times a week or once a week. Some people give themselves the injection; some people get it from their oncology nurse. You may also be instructed to take an iron supplement by mouth while getting these injections.

CARING FOR YOUR SKIN AND HAIR

39. I have heard that radiation therapy causes a skin reaction. Is this true? How should I care for my skin during radiation therapy?

Radiation therapy is administered as a beam of energy directed from a treatment machine at precise angles toward a defined target in your body. It destroys tumor cells in its path by preventing them from dividing. Normal cells that divide rapidly are also very sensitive to the effects of radiation therapy. As a result, there may be changes in your skin where the beam enters and exits your body. After about 2 weeks, you may notice redness, tanning, dryness, flaking, and/or itching. In sensitive areas of the body, such as the armpit and the neck, the reactions may become more severe over time, and you may develop blistering and weeping of the skin. Ask your doctor or nurse to explain what you should expect based on the area being treated. These are all expected effects of radiation, and they will heal about a month after treatment is completed; however, you may be left with an area of darkened skin in the area that was treated.

Take special care of your skin from the first day of treatment to help ensure that you do not become uncomfortable from the changes that occur. Bathe daily using warm water and a mild nonperfumed soap, like Dove®. Do not scrub the skin with a cloth or brush, rinse the skin well to get off all the soap, and gently pat it dry. Your doctor or nurse may recommend use of a moisturizer, for example aloe vera gel or Aquaphor®, either from the beginning of treatment or if you develop dryness or itching. Most commonly, it is recommended to use this twice a day, after your daily treatment and at bedtime. Check before using any other lotions, creams, or ointments in the area being treated, because some products can make the skin reaction more severe.

Take special care of your skin from the first day of treatment.

Avoid irritating the skin in the treated area. Specific suggestions are based on where you are being treated:

- Avoid tight constricting clothing.
- If treatment is to the pelvis, wear cotton underwear.
- Avoid use of tape.
- Avoid scratching the skin. Tell your doctor or nurse if the moisturizers are not effective in relieving the itching so that something else can be prescribed.

- Avoid direct sunlight.
- Avoid use of ice packs or heating pads.

Radiation therapy will also cause the hair in the area being treated to fall out. If you are not being treated to the head or neck area, you will not lose any hair on your head. Your hair will grow back several months after your treatment is completed.

40. I have heard that chemotherapy may cause me to lose my hair. Can I prevent this? What can I do to feel good about my appearance if I lose my hair?

Chemotherapy destroys tumor cells by preventing them from dividing. Normal cells that divide rapidly are very sensitive to the effects of chemotherapy. The cells at the base of the hair follicle may become unable to divide to make new cells, weakening the hair shaft and resulting in loss of hair. Some people experience only a thinning of their hair, but some people lose all of the hair on their head. Certain chemotherapy drugs are much more likely than others to cause hair loss. Your doctor or nurse can tell you if you are likely to lose your hair based on the type of chemotherapy drug that you are receiving. If you are receiving chemotherapy drugs that are likely to cause hair loss, it is also possible that you will lose hair in other parts of your body. Hair anywhere on your body can be affected, including your eyebrows, eyelashes, underarms, and pubic area. Hair loss usually begins about 3 weeks after chemotherapy begins. Sometimes people notice a gradual thinning and loss of hair, but with some chemotherapy agents the hair can come out in clumps over a period of only a few days.

Certain chemotherapy drugs are much more likely than others to cause hair loss.

If you are receiving chemotherapy that causes only a thinning of hair, there are things that may reduce the amount of hair you lose:

- Use a mild shampoo, for example, baby shampoo.
- Use a soft-bristled hairbrush.
- Avoid permanents and hair dyes.
- Avoid heated rollers and high heat hair dryers.

If you are receiving chemotherapy that has a high likelihood of causing complete hair loss, there is no way of preventing this. We no longer use ice caps to prevent the chemotherapy from flowing to the scalp, because we want to be sure the chemotherapy travels all over your body, not missing any area where there could be cancer cells.

If your doctor or nurse tells you there is a high likelihood that you will lose your hair from treatment, you may find it helpful to purchase a wig or hairpiece before you lose your hair. Some people like to match their own hairstyle to maintain their usual appearance. Some people like to try a new look. Wigs can be made with human hair or from synthetic fibers and vary considerably in price. There may be stores in your area that specialize in working with people that lose their hair from cancer treatment, or you can also purchase a wig or hairpiece through the American Cancer Society. Your local American Cancer Society or hospital social work department may also have wigs and hairpieces available to be loaned. When needing a wig or hairpiece because of cancer treatment, your insurance company may reimburse the cost. Check your policy, and if this is covered, ask your doctor to write you a prescription for a "hair prosthesis needed for cancer treatment." Costs that are not reimbursed are tax deductible.

Do whatever makes you feel most comfortable.

Some people prefer to wear a turban, scarf, or cap to cover their head, and some people prefer to leave their head uncovered. Do whatever makes you feel most comfortable. The important thing is to try not to let your changed appearance alter your interactions with family, friends, and coworkers. Despite the loss of hair, there are many things you can do to feel good about your appearance. Taking care in the clothes you wear, using makeup if you like, and wearing beautiful scarves are just some of the ways that may help. In addition, the American Cancer Society and the Cosmetic, Toiletry, and Fragrance Association sponsor a free program, "Look Good, Feel Better," that is dedicated to helping women being treated for cancer feel better about their appearance. They teach beauty techniques that help restore your appearance and enhance your self-image. To find out if it is available in your area, check their Internet site, *www.lookgoodfeelbetter.org*, or call 800-395-LOOK.

41. I have heard there may be changes in the color of my skin from my treatment. What does this mean?

Skin and nail color changes are usually temporary.

Color changes in skin and nails can occur with treatment for cancer. These color changes are usually temporary and can be caused by either chemotherapy or radiation therapy. Changes in skin and nails include

- Flushing;
- Hyperpigmentation;
- Photosensitivity.

Flushing is a temporary redness that usually occurs in the face and neck as a result of capillary dilation. Capillaries are small blood vessels located just under the surface of the skin. Flushing can be caused by chemotherapy (paclitaxel, cisplatin, doxorubicin), intravenous contrast (used with CTs), or some oral medications (steroid medicines such as prednisone or dexamethasone). Alcohol can also cause flushing. Sometimes flushing is accompanied by a feeling of warmth. Flushing is always temporary and generally lasts for minutes or up to several hours.

> **Call your doctor or nurse if the flushing is persistent or is accompanied by pain, fever (100.5°F or more), swelling, or other discomfort.**

Hyperpigmentation is a darkening of the skin; a freckle is an example of hyperpigmentation. This darkening can be generalized, like a suntan, or localized to certain areas of the body. If localized, you may notice darkening of the skin over finger joints or elbows and knees. The palms of the hands and soles of the feet may become darker. There can be a darkening of the tissue under the fingernails and toenails or darkening of the nails themselves. There may even be color changes in your mouth, for example, darkening of your tongue and gums. Certain intravenous chemotherapy (fluorouracil) causes darkening along the length of the vein where it is given. Hyperpigmentation may be more noticeable in people with darker skin tones. Some types of chemotherapy (paclitaxel or docetaxel) cause white lines, called Beau's lines, to form horizontally on the fingernails. Radiation therapy can cause darkening of the skin in the area that is irradiated. Regardless of the cause, exposure to the sun may increase hyperpigmentation temporarily. Hyperpigmentation usually occurs within several days to 2 to 3 weeks after starting treatment. Sometimes the discoloration is permanent, but most often it resolves within a few months after treatment is completed.

Photosensitivity means that your skin is more sensitive to the sun (ultraviolet radiation); you can burn more easily when in the sun or you may develop a rash from the sun. This reaction can occur whether you have light skin or dark skin and may result from medications, including certain types of chemotherapy and antibiotics. Radiation therapy can also cause the skin in the area that was treated to be more sensitive to the sun. Before going out in the sun, ask your doctor or nurse if you are taking any medications that can cause this.

Photosensitivity can result in severe sunburn. This reaction can be prevented. When outside, even on cloudy days, wear protective clothing, including a hat, long-sleeved shirt, and long pants. Always use a sunscreen with an SPF of at least 15 when you are outside. At the beach, sit under an umbrella and use a sunblock such as zinc oxide. If you have had radiation therapy, see Question 39 for additional skin care tips.

If you get a bad sunburn or rash from the sun, call your doctor or nurse. They can prescribe medicines to make you more comfortable. They can also tell you which lotions or creams are best to use for the sunburn.

Lisa's comment:

I am a beach bum—love the summer, love the beach, love the ocean. I have a cabana at Malibu Beach (Long Beach, Long Island). Photosensitivity was probably one of the biggest obstacles for me. I had to wear sunscreen (well, that wasn't new), sit under an umbrella, and not go in the ocean (that wasn't because of chemotherapy, but because of surgery restrictions). I felt like my one true pleasure was a chore, a burden. I did very well with keeping myself protected from the sun, but I really didn't entirely enjoy my days at the beach. But, chemotherapy didn't stop me from going!! My fingernails turned a yellowish-orange color with the Adriamycin/Cytoxan therapy.

42. I have heard that some chemotherapy drugs can burn your skin. What does this mean?

Most chemotherapy drugs are given through a vein. Oncology nurses generally receive special training on techniques to administer these drugs safely and accurately. Despite using the most careful technique, the drugs can sometimes leak out of the veins and collect under the skin. With most chemotherapy, the body reabsorbs the fluid with no ill effects. However, some chemotherapy drugs can cause blistering and may damage the skin and the underlying tissues if they leak out of the vein (**extravasation**). These are called **vesicants**; examples include cisplatin, doxorubicin, vincristine, and paclitaxel. Other chemotherapy drugs may cause irritation and inflammation if they leak under the skin but will not cause any tissue damage.

Extravasation

a potential complication of intravenous chemotherapy administration that occurs when chemotherapy leaks from the vein into the surrounding tissue.

Vesicants

chemotherapy that causes blistering or other local tissue damage if it leaks from a vein into the surrounding tissue. Only some types of chemotherapy are classified as vesicants.

If you feel pain or burning while your nurse is giving you treatment, let him or her know right away. If there is any indication that chemotherapy has leaked out of the vein, the nurse will stop the treatment and remove the needle. If the chemotherapy is a vesicant, the nurse may apply hot or cold compresses or may inject or apply special medicine to the area. Keep an eye on the site over the next 2 weeks. Very rarely, serious reactions can develop. Call your doctor or nurse if you have pain, if the area becomes red or swollen, or if you see blisters

If you feel pain or burning while your nurse is giving you treatment, let him or her know right away.

or ulcers. They will reevaluate you and refer you to a plastic surgeon if necessary.

Lisa's comment:

I wanted a mediport as soon as I heard I would need chemotherapy. I had always told my patients: "If I were to get chemo, I would get a mediport." I said it because I meant it. Being diagnosed with breast cancer and requiring an axillary node dissection meant I only had one arm available for intravenous therapy. I knew I was scheduled to receive Adriamycin/Paclitaxel—vesicants (medications given by vein). So, I really wanted a mediport. I guess deep down I didn't trust anyone to give me chemotherapy. Needless to say, the Breast Service didn't recommend port placement for only eight cycles of chemotherapy—not worth the surgical risks. I did fine. The nurses did not have trouble with my veins and I never had an extravasation (a "blown" or leaky vein).

43. What is jaundice and how can it be treated?

Bilirubin is produced when the liver breaks down hemoglobin, the oxygen-carrying substance in red blood cells. It is then incorporated into the bile, giving it a yellow-green color. Bile is stored in the gallbladder, and after eating the gallbladder pushes the bile out through the bile duct into the intestine where it digests certain types of food. It is then eliminated in the stool. Bilirubin helps to give stool its usual brown color.

If bilirubin builds up in the bloodstream, it lodges in the skin and eyes, causing them to become yellow in color. This is referred to as jaundice (or icterus). Some of this excess bilirubin will be eliminated in the urine, causing it to become darker in color. If the bilirubin is not able to pass into the intestine, the stools become lighter in color.

There are a number of reasons people with cancer may develop increased bilirubin and jaundice: either not enough bilirubin is being eliminated or too much bilirubin is being produced. A mass in the bile duct or in the area around the duct (for example, in the gall-bladder, liver, or pancreas) may block the flow of bile though the duct, interfering with the elimination of bilirubin. Disease in the liver may also reduce the body's ability to eliminate bilirubin. Certain blood disorders in which a large number of red blood cells are destroyed may cause increased levels of bilirubin.

Sometimes jaundice can be treated. If the bile duct is blocked in a localized area, a small hollow tube can be inserted to open up the duct, relieving the obstruction. If the liver disease or blood disorder is treatable, the bilirubin will come down. However, if the jaundice cannot be treated, there are ways to ensure you are comfortable.

Jaundice itself causes no pain; however, the skin may become very dry and itchy. Scratching may create breaks in the skin, which could become infected, so preventing itching is important. Treating the dryness will help reduce the itching. When bathing, avoid very hot water and use only mild soaps. Apply skin lotions or creams after bathing and throughout the day as needed to moisturize the skin. If you still feel itchy, ask your doctor for a prescription for medication that will reduce the itching. See Question 30 for additional tips on how to control itching.

44. What do I do if I get a rash?

A rash is a skin reaction that may be localized to one area of the body or it may cover most or all of the body (generalized). Rashes are most commonly caused by medications; they can be a side effect of the medicine (for example, causing an acne-like rash) or can be a sign of an allergic reaction. Rashes can also be caused by an illness such as a virus; measles and shingles are examples of viruses. A rash can also be caused by a change in laundry detergent, moisturizer, or soap. Rashes may cause some discomfort like itching or pain.

If you develop a rash, call your doctor or nurse.

If you develop a rash, call your doctor or nurse. Be prepared to tell where the rash is located, what the rash looks like, when it started, and if there are any other symptoms such as fever, itching, or pain. Tell them if you have recently started using a new medicine. Words that can be used to describe a rash include raised (bumpy), flat, or blisters. Describe the color, for example, red, purplish, or skin colored.

Antihistamine
medication that is used to prevent or treat allergic reactions; it is sometimes given to treat itching caused by a rash.

If there is itching associated with the rash, your doctor may prescribe diphenhydramine, an **antihistamine** that can be bought over the counter. This may make you sleepy and give you a dry mouth. Your doctor may also prescribe calamine lotion for an itchy rash. Taking a bath with Aveeno or oatmeal may be soothing. If your doctor thinks that your rash is an allergic reaction to medicine that you are taking, he or she may tell you to stop taking the medicine. If your doctor thinks your rash is from shingles, he or she will prescribe an antiviral medicine. See Question 45 for more information about shingles.

If your rash is associated with hives or difficulty breathing, call your doctor and go to the nearest emergency room.

45. What is shingles?

Shingles (herpes zoster) is caused by the same virus that causes chicken pox. You can only get shingles if you have had chicken pox in the past, and about 1 in 10 people who have had chicken pox will get shingles. This infection is more common if you are 60 years or older and are getting treatment for cancer.

Once you have had chicken pox, the virus stays in your body and hibernates, remaining inactive, in the nerve cells along your spine. If the virus becomes active, it will travel along a nerve tract on one side of your body. This can cause tingling, a burning type pain, itching, and a blister-like rash following a line or band on the skin over the involved nerve. Very often, the pain and itching start 1 to 4 days before you can see the rash. If you develop a rash (not everyone does), the blisters are small and tear-shaped. Shingles can occur anywhere on the body but most often occurs on the chest or back.

Shingles itself is not contagious (catching). However, if you have shingles, you can give chicken pox to someone who has not had chicken pox before. Your blisters will crust over and dry up in about 7 to 10 days. Once this happens, you are no longer contagious. Sometimes people continue to have pain even when the rash goes away. This is called **postherpetic neuralgia**.

If you think that you have shingles, call your doctor or nurse. Your doctor will prescribe an antiviral medicine

Postherpetic neuralgia

localized pain that occurs in the area where shingles was present.

Blood Counts and Skin Problems

83

(for example, acyclovir, famciclovir). This medicine can be taken as a pill, given through a vein (intravenously), or applied as a cream on the blisters. You will need to take this medicine several times a day for 7 to 10 days. It is important to take this medicine just as the doctor tells you to. If you develop postherpetic neuralgia, your doctor will prescribe pain medicine. This pain medicine may be taken as a pill, or sometimes a cream is rubbed into the skin where the rash was located. If this medicine doesn't help your pain, follow up with your doctor.

> **Call your doctor if you**
> - **Think you have shingles;**
> - **Have shingles near your eye;**
> - **Have a rash with a fever of 100.5°F or more.**

PART FIVE

Problems with Breathing, Nutrition, Digestion, and Urination

I feel short of breath. What can I do
to ease my breathing?

What can I do to increase
my appetite and maintain my weight?

What can I do to manage nausea and vomiting?

What can I do to manage constipation?

What can I do for incontinence?

More . . .

46. I feel short of breath. What can I do to ease my breathing?

When people feel short of breath, they describe this as having difficulty breathing or a feeling that they cannot get enough air. Some people say they feel "winded." **Dyspnea** is the medical term that describes this feeling. In people who have cancer, shortness of breath can be caused by the cancer, by treatment for cancer, or it may be unrelated to cancer. Some causes of shortness of breath are as follows:

Dyspnea

difficult or labored breathing; shortness of breath.

- Lung damage from cancer, radiation therapy, chemotherapy, or lung surgery
- Blood clots in the lung (also called **pulmonary embolism**)
- Fluid build up around the heart or lungs (called pericardial or pleural effusions)
- Lung infection
- Heart failure (called congestive heart failure)
- Asthma and emphysema (also known as chronic obstructive pulmonary disease, or COPD)
- Anemia (see Question 38)
- Stress or anxiety

Pulmonary embolism

a blood clot in the lung. A pulmonary embolism usually starts when a blood clot travels from a vein in the legs to the pulmonary artery; this can cause sudden shortness of breath.

The best way to relieve shortness of breath is to treat its cause. Even if the condition is not treatable or the cause is unknown, measures can be taken to help you breathe better. If you have shortness of breath, talk to your doctor or nurse. They will work with you to determine the best way to improve your breathing.

Measures can be taken to help you breathe better.

Your doctor may prescribe medicine to treat your shortness of breath: inhalers for asthma or emphysema, antibiotics for infection, epoetin for anemia, or blood thinners for a blood clot. If it is determined that your shortness of breath is caused by stress or anxiety, an antianxiety medicine such as lorazepam may be prescribed. Other medicines that are sometimes used include corticosteroids and the pain medicine, morphine. Morphine helps people to breathe better by slowing the breathing rate, which allows people to take deeper more effective breaths. If the doctor prescribes medicine for your shortness of breath, do not stop taking it unless you have your doctor's approval.

There are other nondrug measures that can help people who have shortness of breath. If you have low oxygen in your blood, your doctor will prescribe oxygen (see Question 47). Sometimes acupuncture or acupressure can help to relieve shortness of breath. Your doctor or nurse can refer you to someone who performs acupressure or acupuncture. Some breathing exercises, such as diaphragmatic breathing, can help people decrease shortness of breath. These breathing exercises will also help you to take slower more effective breaths. Ask your nurse to provide you with instructions for diaphragmatic breathing exercises.

If you have shortness of breath, you may be more comfortable sitting up and using pillows for support. Reclining chairs are helpful for sleeping and allow you to be in a semi-sitting position. Schedule rest periods at regular intervals during activities to relieve shortness of breath. Sometimes an open window or a fan in the room is helpful.

> **Call your doctor or nurse if you have the following:**
> - **Sudden difficulty breathing or inability to catch your breath**
> - **Worsening shortness of breath despite the treatments given to you**

- **Discomfort or pain in the chest when breathing**
- **Bloody or discolored phlegm (also called sputum)**
- **Difficulty sleeping when lying down**
- **Fever of 100.5°F or more**

47. How do I know if I need oxygen?

Oxygen is essential for cells to function normally in the body. Not all shortness of breath is caused by low oxygen. To test for low oxygen, a small device called a pulse oximeter is placed on your finger. If it shows that you have a low oxygen level, your doctor will prescribe oxygen. Your doctor will determine the amount of oxygen (referred to as liters of oxygen) you need.

Oxygen can be provided for you at home. It is supplied by a respiratory or home care company. Oxygen comes in different types of containers. There are cylinders that contain oxygen. Alternatively, a small machine that pulls oxygen from room air can be set up at home; this is plugged into an electrical outlet. The oxygen travels through a tube that extends from the unit. This tube is attached to another tube (called a nasal cannula) that is placed in your nostrils. Smaller portable units are also available that are easier to use outside the house. Oxygen may be covered by your health insurance provider.

Great care must be used when oxygen is in the home.

Great care must be used when oxygen is in the home. Oxygen itself is nonflammable; however, materials will burn more readily in the presence of increased oxygen. When oxygen is not in use, the container should be turned off. Under no circumstances should matches, lighters, cigarettes, or candles be used in the room where oxygen is used or stored. Additionally, oxygen containers should not be stored near gas or electrical heating elements. Your respiratory therapist or the company that provides the oxygen will review other safety measures with you and your family or caregivers.

48. What should I do if I cough up blood?

If you cough up blood, you should call your doctor or nurse. Coughing up blood from the lower respiratory tract (below the throat) or lungs is called **hemoptysis**. Sometimes the phlegm (sputum) is tinged or streaked with blood, and at other times people cough up bright red blood. If possible, estimate the amount of blood that has been coughed up (for example, one tablespoon, one-half cup) and note the color (for example, bright red, dark, like coffee grounds).

If you cough up blood, call your doctor or nurse.

Hemoptysis
spitting up blood or blood-tinged sputum.

There are many causes of hemoptysis, and the most common cause is infection such as bronchitis. In some instances, cancer can also cause hemoptysis. Other causes include a blood clot in the lung, tuberculosis, heart problems, and pneumonia. Sometimes it is difficult to tell if the blood is coming from the lungs, back of the mouth, or stomach (vomiting of blood or hematemesis). Telling the doctor about other symptoms that you have and the color of the blood can help him or her to make a diagnosis.

The doctor may also order certain tests such as a complete blood count (CBC) (analyzes the different components of the blood) or **coagulation profile** (analyzes the clotting ability of the blood). He or she may also want a specimen of your sputum to determine whether infection is present. A chest x-ray or CT (commonly referred to as a "CAT" scan) may reveal abnormalities in the lungs. And the doctor may want to look at your lungs and air passages directly through a scope (bronchoscopy).

Coagulation profile
a blood test that analyzes the clotting ability of the blood.

Treatment of hemoptysis depends on the cause and the amount of blood that is coughed up. When hemoptysis is mild and infection is suspected, antibiotics are usually prescribed. In addition to antibiotics, a cough suppressant (codeine) is prescribed, because coughing can cause irritation and can aggravate hemoptysis. For most patients, the conservative measures listed above usually stop the problem.

NUTRITIONAL PROBLEMS

49. I never feel hungry and am concerned about losing weight. What can I do to increase my appetite and maintain my weight?

Weight loss is a common problem for people with cancer. This can occur for many reasons. Having cancer changes your metabolism, so you need more calories each day than you usually consume. You may find you have a poor appetite or a feeling of being full after eating only a few bites of food. Food may taste differently, and symptoms such as nausea, gas, constipation, pain, fatigue, or emotional distress can further decrease your appetite. Changes in your mouth from the disease or treatment may make it difficult to chew and swallow adequate amounts of nutrients and fluids. And finally, changes in how your body digests or absorbs food may make it difficult for you to use the nutrients and fluids you are able to take in.

It is important to eat and drink adequate amounts of food and fluids to provide energy to your body and help you better tolerate your treatment. Try to maintain your usual weight or minimize the amount of weight you lose. Even if you are overweight when you begin treatment, it is generally not recommended to diet at this time. There are a number of things you can do to improve your appetite and help maintain your weight.

Medication may be helpful if you have symptoms that are affecting your appetite, like mouth sores, nausea, vomiting, diarrhea, constipation, pain, or emotional distress. If you have any of these problems, ask your doctor for medication to help with these.

Make changes in your diet to maximize the amount of nutrients you take in each day. Suggestions include the following:

- Eat small amounts of food and fluids at a time. Eat six or eight snacks throughout the day rather than trying to eat three full meals. Always have food nearby to nibble on.
- Select foods high in protein and calories. Foods that many people find easy to eat when they are not very hungry include
  - Eggs;
  - Cottage cheese or yogurt;
  - Peanut butter;
  - Sandwiches with sliced turkey or tuna fish;
  - Baked or broiled chicken, fish, or beef;
  - Soups.
- Add a variety of things to recipes to add calories, for example, butter, honey, jelly, sour cream, cheese, yogurt, cream, and evaporated milk. *Eating Hints for Cancer Patients*, published by the National Cancer Institute, provides many helpful recipes.
- Limit the amount of fluids you take with your meals so that you don't fill up on the fluid.
- Have a limited amount of beverages with caffeine (for example, coffee, tea, many sodas) because these will dehydrate you.

Select foods high in protein and calories.

91

- Have a limited amount of carbonated beverages, because they will make you feel full.
- Replace fluids with no nutritional benefit, like water or soda, with fluids that provide nutrients, like cream soups, shakes, and fruit smoothies.
- Try nutritional supplements that are available in your local drugstore. These may be canned drinks, powders to be mixed with water or milk, or puddings. Experiment with different brands to find products you enjoy. Your doctor or nurse may recommend specific supplements for you. You can also use Carnation Instant Breakfast®, blending it with milk and adding ice cream, yogurt, and/or fruit.

Other suggestions that may be helpful are as follows:

- Ask your doctor or nurse if it is safe for you to have a glass of wine or beer or a cocktail before your meal. Many people find that alcohol stimulates their appetite.
- Avoid eating alone. Having company can make eating more enjoyable, and we often eat more when eating with someone else.
- See Question 50 for suggestions to improve your intake of food and fluid if you are having problems related to changes in taste and Question 52 for suggestions if you are having problems related to swallowing.

It is common for family members and friends to have suggestions and want to give you advice. They may recommend special diets, high-protein drinks, or supplemental megavitamins and antioxidants. Do not take these without first speaking with your doctor or nurse as they may interfere with your treatment or may be dangerous for you.

It is often frustrating for family members who work hard to prepare special foods only to have you push it away after only a few bites. Avoid conflicts, but remind them that you are only able to eat what your appetite allows. Eating should be pleasurable; eat what you want when you want it. You may find it helpful to speak with a nutritionist for guidance in what to eat. These are registered dietitians, certified by the American Dietetic Association. Ask your doctor or nurse for a referral to a nutritionist with expertise in working with people who have cancer.

> **Call your doctor if you are unable to eat or drink for more than a day for any reason.**

50. Nothing tastes the way it used to, and sometimes I have an awful taste in my mouth. What can I do for this?

Pete's comment:

I have been on chemotherapy for over a year. For several days following treatment, most food tastes very bland and unappetizing. I also have the sensation of feeling slightly queasy. For this period, I have changed my diet to include spicy foods, drink plenty of ginger ale, switch from coffee to tea and eat smaller more frequent meals. This approach has enabled me to maintain my weight and actually get more variety into my diet. I also take Prilosec twice a day to help digestion.

Changes in the way food tastes and smells can be caused by certain medicines (for example, antibiotics), some types of chemotherapy, radiation therapy to the head and neck, and surgery in the mouth or head and neck area. The cancer itself can also cause changes in taste. This can be a problem, because it may cause you to decrease your food intake, lose weight, or develop a food aversion (a strong dislike for a certain food). If you are getting treatment for your cancer, it is important that you maintain your weight and maintain good nutrition.

Most people have four taste sensations: salty, sweet, bitter, and sour. These may be exaggerated by treatment for your cancer, making foods taste differently than they normally would. In addition, some people note a persistent metallic or bitter taste, and some people note a lack of taste or no taste. These changes can be worse if you have a dry mouth (see Question 53 for tips on handling a dry mouth) or a change in your sense of smell. Chemotherapy medicines that most often cause alterations in taste include cisplatin, cyclophosphamide, doxorubicin, fluorouracil, paclitaxel, and vincristine. For most people, these changes in taste are temporary and will go away when the treatment is finished; however, this may take weeks to months.

One of the most important things you can do is maintain good oral hygiene.

There are several things you can try to improve the flavor of the food you eat. One of the most important things you can do is maintain good oral hygiene. This includes brushing your teeth on a regular basis and using a mouthwash four to five times a day. Rinsing your mouth immediately before eating to moisten the taste buds on your tongue is particularly helpful. Some people use a solution of baking soda and water; others use a commercial mouthwash like Biotene. Do not use a mouthwash that contains alcohol because it causes dryness and may worsen the problem. Your doctor or nurse can recommend a mouth care regimen. You can also ask your dentist for recommendations.

There are several other things you can do to enhance your appetite and the flavor of your food. First, always eat foods that look and smell good to you. If you have an aversion to the smell of food, ask a family member to cook or grill outdoors for you. Use a fan in the kitchen to eliminate or reduce cooking odors. Eat foods that are cold or at room temperature to reduce the smell. If food has a metallic taste, use plastic utensils to prepare and eat food. Try marinating or basting meat or poultry with fruit juices or wine to improve their taste. If food is bland, add herbs or other seasonings to enhance the flavor. For more suggestions, the National Cancer Institute has a booklet entitled *Eating Hints for Cancer Patients*. This booklet addresses changes in sense of taste and smell as well as management of other eating problems. It is available on the Internet at *cancer.gov/cancerinfo/eatinghints*. You can also order this booklet over the phone by calling the Cancer Information Service. Your doctor or nurse can help suggest other eating hints or refer you to a registered dietitian.

Some studies have shown that taking zinc can improve the taste of food in people who had radiotherapy to the head and neck area. Zinc may also be beneficial in people getting other treatments for cancer. Before taking any medication to improve the flavor of food or enhance your appetite, including zinc, check with your doctor or nurse.

51. I have heard that my treatment may cause sores in my mouth. How should I care for my mouth during chemotherapy?

Pete's comment:

Right from the start, I was worried about mouth sores. I switched to Biotene mouthwash which I use in the morn-

ing and evening. I also continue to brush my teeth three or four times a day and drink plenty of fluids. Fortunately, I have been free of mouth sores since starting treatment.

Chemotherapy and radiation therapy destroy tumor cells by preventing them from dividing. Normal cells that divide rapidly are also sensitive to the effects of these treatments. With certain chemotherapy drugs and with radiation therapy to the head and neck region, the mucous membranes lining the inside of your mouth and throat may be affected. They may become reddened and may feel tender, sore, or painful. You may even develop sores or ulcers in the mouth or throat or have difficulty swallowing. This is called **stomatitis**. Some chemotherapy drugs are much more likely than others to cause mouth sores. If you develop severe mouth sores, your doctor may reduce the dose of chemotherapy for your next treatment.

Stomatitis

inflammation or irritation of the mucous membranes in the mouth; this can be caused by chemotherapy or radiation therapy.

Keep your mouth clean and moist to prevent infection.

Keep your mouth clean and moist to prevent infection. Brush your teeth with a soft-bristled toothbrush after each meal and rinse regularly with a saltwater solution to keep your mouth moist. Add a teaspoon of table salt or baking soda to a glass of warm water to swish and spit. Do not use any commercial mouthwash that contains alcohol because this can irritate your mouth.

If you wear dentures that are not fitting correctly, you will be more likely to get sores in your mouth from the rubbing and irritation of the dentures. This may be a problem, particularly if you have lost weight recently; your gums may have shrunk, changing the fit of your dentures. If you are unsure about the fit of your dentures, see your dentist to adjust them if needed.

If you have sores in your mouth or throat, the membranes may become infected. This is most commonly caused by candida, a type of fungus. Your mouth may look very red, and you may see white, cheesy-looking patches on the membranes or tongue. If you notice these, call your doctor or nurse so they can examine you and prescribe an antibiotic if you do have an infection.

See Question 52 for suggestions on how to manage pain from mouth sores and on how to ensure you eat and drink enough even if you have pain with swallowing.

> **Call your doctor if you are unable to eat or drink for more than a day because of painful mouth sores or if you develop white, cheesy-looking patches in your mouth.**

52. My mouth and throat hurt, and swallowing food and liquid is difficult or painful. What can I do to help with this?

Swallowing food and liquid may be difficult or painful for a variety of reasons. A tumor in the mouth, throat, or esophagus or surgery in this area may alter the muscles and other tissues or may cause a blockage in the pathways involved in swallowing. If you are getting chemotherapy or radiation therapy to the head and neck region or chest, you can develop irritation or sores on the mucous membranes lining the inside of your mouth, throat, or esophagus (see Question 51). Certain medications like steroids may increase your risk of developing an infection in your mouth, particularly with candida, a type of fungus, which may cause pain when you swallow.

Changes in what you eat and drink may be helpful

If you are having pain or difficulty when you swallow, changes in what you eat and drink may be helpful:

- Eat soft or pureed foods that are easy to chew and swallow.
- If you are having difficulty swallowing solid foods, drink liquid nutritional supplements that are available in your local drugstore. Experiment with different brands to find products you enjoy. Your doctor or nurse may recommend specific supplements for you.
- If you are having difficulty swallowing fluids, try thick cream soups, shakes, fruit smoothies, jell-o, ice cream, and frozen juices to be sure you get enough liquid during the day.
- Avoid hot foods or liquids.
- Avoid foods and liquids that can irritate the membranes such as alcohol, citrus, tomatoes, spices, and rough coarse foods.
- Avoid smoking.

Swallowing will be painful if your mouth or throat becomes sore or painful. Let your doctor or nurse know so something can be prescribed for you. A variety of medications may be used, including topical anesthetic medications you can swish in your mouth to numb the membranes (for example, lidocaine), products that coat the membranes to protect them (for example, GelClair), and combination mouthwashes (sometimes called "magic mouthwash"). If your mouth is very painful, a narcotic medication may be needed. If your lips become irritated, vitamin A&D ointment can be soothing.

If you are having difficulty swallowing your medications, ask your doctor to prescribe a liquid version if it is available. If there is not a liquid version available, many medications can be crushed and mixed with a small amount of juice or applesauce to make them easier to swallow. Check with your pharmacist before crushing any medication because this may affect the way the medication works.

If you are unable to swallow enough food and fluid to maintain your weight, your doctor may recommend that you get a **feeding tube**. This is placed through the wall of your abdomen directly into the stomach. Liquid nutritional supplements are instilled through the tube every few hours throughout the day. You can get all the nutrients and fluids you need through a feeding tube.

Feeding tube
a tube placed through the abdominal wall into the stomach; this is used to give liquid nutritional supplements.

> **Call your doctor if you are unable to eat or drink for more than a day because of pain or difficulty swallowing.**

53. What can I do for my dry mouth?

Dry mouth (xerostomia) occurs when the glands that make saliva don't work effectively. This can result from radiation therapy or surgery to the head and neck area, certain chemotherapy drugs, certain medications (for example, many of the medications used to treat high blood pressure and depression, antihistamines, and decongestants), and certain medical problems like diabetes, Parkinson's disease, Sjögren's disease, and HIV or AIDS. If you don't have enough saliva or spit to keep your mouth moist, you may have an uncomfortable dry feeling in your mouth and throat, you may have changes in your sense of taste, it may be difficult to chew and swallow food, and you may even find it difficult to speak. A loss of saliva can also cause increased dental decay and an increased chance of developing infections in your mouth.

There are a number of things you can do to help manage a dry mouth:

- Keep your mouth moist. Take frequent small sips of liquids throughout the day and suck on ice cubes of frozen water or juice.
- Use a saliva substitute like Biotene Oral Balance Moisturizing Gel.
- Avoid tobacco, alcohol, and caffeine, all of which can dry the mouth.
- Take sips of fluids while eating and moisten foods with gravy, sauce, broth, or yogurt to make them easier to swallow.
- Try to stimulate the glands to produce more saliva by chewing sugar-free gum or sucking on sugar-free hard candies.
- Ask your doctor about medications that can help stimulate more saliva. If your glands are able to produce saliva but are not working properly, medication such as pilocarpine may help.

Avoid tobacco, alcohol, and caffeine, all of which can dry the mouth.

To prevent dental decay, brush your teeth after each meal using fluoride toothpaste. It is important to see a dentist regularly because of your increased risk for dental decay. Your dentist may recommend a fluoride gel to use at night.

For additional information, the National Oral Health Information Clearinghouse of the National Institutes of Health provides a free publication, *Dry Mouth*, available on the Internet at *www.nohic.nidcr.nih.gov/pubs/drymouth/dmouth.htm#1* or by calling 301-496-4261.

DIGESTIVE PROBLEMS

54. What can I do to help with heartburn?

Heartburn is a sensation of burning in the chest, most commonly felt behind the breastbone. Some people describe a sensation that food or liquid is coming back up into the throat, and some describe an acid or bitter taste in the back of their throat, "acid indigestion." Heartburn has nothing to do with the heart and is actually caused by a backflow, or reflux, of the digestive stomach acids into the esophagus where they cause irritation of the lining of the esophagus.

The most common cause of heartburn is GERD, gastroesophageal reflux disease. This develops when the muscle at the lower end of the esophagus does not work properly. This muscle is in the form of a ring, or sphincter. The muscle opens to allow food to pass from the esophagus into the stomach; at other times it tightens and stays closed to prevent stomach contents from flowing backward into the esophagus. If the muscle does not close properly, there is reflux resulting in symptoms of heartburn.

Heartburn may also be caused by increased pressure on the stomach. This may be from excess weight or from a tumor or fluid in the abdomen or pelvis pushing up against the stomach. Other causes include certain medications, foods and fluids that increase the acidity of the stomach, and hiatal hernia (a weakening of the diaphragm muscle causing part of the stomach to rise into the chest).

There are a number of steps you can take to treat heartburn; however, if you have heartburn lasting more than 2 weeks or occurring more than two

Call your doctor if heartburn lasts more than 2 weeks or occurs more than twice a week.

times a week, call your doctor. If untreated, reflux can cause serious problems, such as ulceration in the esophagus, scarring and narrowing of the esophagus, and even changes in the cells of the membranes lining the esophagus that put them at risk of developing into a cancer.

Changes in your diet are helpful. Avoid foods that are known to bring on heartburn: citrus, tomatoes, onions, garlic, fatty foods, mint, and pepper. Avoid caffeinated, alcoholic, carbonated, and citrus beverages that may also bring on heartburn. Have small portions of food at a time and do not eat at bedtime.

Positioning also plays a role. Sit upright when eating and drinking and do not lie down or bend over at the waist for at least 2 hours after eating a meal. Elevate the head of the bed 6 to 8 inches if you have symptoms when lying down. Avoid wearing clothes that are tight around the belly, and if you wear a belt, keep it loosely closed.

A variety of medications is helpful in treating heartburn. Some are available over the counter and some require a prescription. Antacids are salts of aluminum, magnesium, calcium, or a combination of these, which neutralize acid. They work quickly but only last up to 2 hours. Histamine receptor antagonists (H_2 blockers) reduce the production of acid by blocking histamine, one of the chemicals that stimulate the stomach to make acid. These generally take about 30 to 60 minutes to work and may last up to 10 hours. H_2 blockers include cimetidine, ranitidine, famotidine, and nizatidine. Proton pump inhibitors (PPIs) reduce the production of acid by blocking the pump that makes the acid.

PPIs include omeprazole, lansoprazole, and esomeprazole. These generally take about 60 minutes to work but may last up to 24 hours. H_2 blockers and PPIs may be used regularly to prevent problems. Before taking any medication, ask your doctor or nurse which medication is best for you, how much to take, and how often to take it. The Heartburn Alliance has additional information on this problem at *www.heartburnalliance.org*.

55. I have heard that radiation therapy or chemotherapy may cause nausea and vomiting. What can I do to manage these symptoms?

Lisa's comment:

I was lucky not to experience the classic "nausea or vomiting" side effect associated with chemotherapy. However, my gastrointestinal side effects manifested with a "heavy gut" feeling—I felt like I swallowed a bunch of rocks. It would start the day after treatment and last about three days. By my fourth cycle of therapy, the feeling would start the night before (anticipatory). Eating helped my symptoms somewhat. I was on so many anti-nausea drugs, I could not help think that my symptoms were related to them. All and all, I figured it was better to have the "heavy gut" rather than the actual nausea and/or vomiting. I could tolerate these symptoms because I knew once I got off the adriamycin/cyclophosphamide, the paclitaxel would be easier to tolerate.

Nausea and vomiting have long been considered to be unavoidable side effects of cancer treatment. However, with the development in recent years of new anti-nausea medications (**antiemetics**), this is no longer the case.

Antiemetics
medication used to prevent or treat nausea and vomiting.

103

Radiation therapy to the abdominal area and a variety of chemotherapy drugs may cause nausea or vomiting. This can result from irritation of the stomach or from chemical stimulation of areas in the brain that trigger nausea and vomiting. Nausea is often experienced as feeling sick to your stomach or feeling queasy. Vomiting is when you throw up stomach contents through your mouth. Retching, gagging, or dry heaves feel similar to vomiting, but no stomach contents come up.

People vary widely in their reactions to the same treatment. Some people have very distressing nausea or vomiting, some have mild symptoms, and some have none at all. For people who do experience nausea or vomiting, the timing of the symptoms will also vary. Some people develop symptoms within minutes or hours after treatment and some develop symptoms days later. For some people the symptoms last several hours, and for others they persist for many days. For some people, the most severe symptoms occur before leaving home in the morning or while on the way to treatment; this is called "anticipatory" nausea or vomiting.

Of the many effective ways of managing nausea and vomiting, most important is the use of medication. See Question 56 for a review of the medications available.

There are also ways to manage nausea or vomiting that do not rely on medication. There are techniques using your body and mind that can be very helpful, particularly with anticipatory nausea or vomiting. Examples include guided imagery, self-hypnosis, and progressive muscle relaxation. If you are interested in learning one of these techniques, ask your doctor or nurse for a referral to someone trained in this field. Another helpful strategy is to minimize the use of things in the home that have particularly strong odors, like perfumes or certain cleaning products.

Changes in what you eat and drink may also help in managing nausea and vomiting. Some specific suggestions include:

- Eat a light meal before each treatment.
- Eat small amounts of food and liquids at a time.
- Eat bland foods and liquids.
- Eat dry crackers when feeling nauseated.
- Limit the amount of liquids you take with your meals.
- Maintain adequate liquids in between meals; take mostly clear liquids such as water, apple juice, herbal tea, or bouillon. Some people find that carbonated sodas are helpful; others do better drinking soda without the fizz.
- Eat cool foods or foods at room temperature.
- Avoid foods with strong odors.
- Avoid high fat, greasy, and fried foods.
- Avoid spicy foods, alcohol, and caffeine.

Taking in adequate amounts of fluids and nutrients is important for your health. If you feel that seeing a nutritionist would help you in selecting appropriate foods, ask your doctor or nurse for a referral. For additional information on managing nausea and vomiting, the National Comprehensive Cancer Network has guidelines for patients at *www.nccn.org*.

> **Call your doctor or nurse if you are unable to keep any food or fluids down for 12 hours, or if you are taking in only minimal amounts for 24 hours.**

56. What medications are available to treat nausea and vomiting?

There are a number of medications available to treat nausea and vomiting, and several new medications have recently been developed. As we have learned new ways of using and combining these medications, nausea and vomiting can be prevented or well controlled in most people. Anti-nausea medications are called antiemetics.

These medications are most commonly given orally, intravenously, or by rectal suppository. Depending on the specific treatment you are getting, and on the timing and severity of your symptoms, your doctor will prescribe a specific anti-nausea medication for you. You may be instructed to take the medication at home before coming for treatment, the nurse may give you medication immediately before your chemotherapy, or you may be instructed to take the medication on a schedule at home after your treatment. Sometimes, depending on the type of treatment you are getting, your doctor will give you a combination of two or three medicines. For example, if you are getting chemotherapy that is likely to cause moderate to severe nausea or vomiting, your doctor may prescribe one or two medications for the nurse to give you before your treatment and medications for you to take at home after treatment. Different anti-nausea medications work in different ways, so if one medication is not effective, call your doctor or nurse and ask for something else to take. Below are some of the medications most commonly used to treat nausea and vomiting related to cancer or cancer treatment. In addition, lorazepam (Ativan) can be given either intravenously or by mouth if you experience anticipatory nausea.

Medication	How taken
For Moderate to Severe Nausea and Vomiting	
Granisetron (Kytril)	Tablet or IV
Ondansetron (Zofran)	Tablet or IV
Palonosetron (Aloxi)	IV
Aprepitant (Emend)	Tablet
Dolasetron (Anzemet)	Tablet or IV
Dexamethasone (Decadron)	Tablet or IV
For Mild Nausea	
Prochlorperazine (Compazine)	Tablet, Injection, or Suppository
Metoclopramide (Reglan)	Tablet or Injection

Many of these medications can cause constipation. See Question 58 on tips to manage constipation.

> Nausea and vomiting can be effectively treated; let your doctor or nurse know if you are having persistent symptoms.

57. I have heard that radiation therapy or chemotherapy may cause diarrhea. What can I do to treat these symptoms?

Chemotherapy and radiation therapy destroy tumor cells by preventing them from dividing. Normal cells that divide rapidly are also very sensitive to the effects of these treatments. Certain chemotherapy drugs and radiation to the abdominal or pelvic area will cause the mucous membranes lining the small intestine to become thinner and lose their ability to function as effectively as normal. As a result, the intestines do not absorb fluid and nutrients adequately and do not digest lactose (the sugar in milk) well. In addition, the muscle layer of the intestine may become overactive, moving the intestinal contents through the bowel more quickly than usual. All of this may result in abdominal cramping and diarrhea. Some chemotherapy drugs are much more likely than others to cause diarrhea.

There are many effective ways of managing cramping and diarrhea. Antidiarrheal medications such as loperamide (Imodium AD, over the counter) or Lomotil (requires a prescription) are very effective. Your doctor or nurse will instruct you on how to take these medications.

Changes in what you eat and drink will also help in managing diarrhea. Some specific suggestions are as follows:

- Eat small amounts of food and liquids at a time.
- Eat bland foods and liquids.
- Increase the amount of fluid you drink when having diarrhea.
- Drink a variety of liquids, selecting clear liquids you can see through like apple juice, cranberry juice, herbal teas, and Jell-o.
- Sports drinks with electrolytes are particularly good to take, as well as fat-free broth or bouillon.
- Eat bananas, applesauce, canned cooked fruits with skin removed, white potatoes without the skin, cooked squash or carrots, and tomato paste or puree (without chunks of tomato). Bananas and white potatoes are good sources of potassium, which is important to replace when having diarrhea.
- Avoid liquids with alcohol and caffeine.
- Avoid high-fiber foods.

- Avoid whole grain breads and cereals. Instead have white bread, pasta, noodles, cold cereals of corn or rice, saltines, and white rice.
- Avoid raw fruits (except bananas) and vegetables, cooked vegetables that cause gas, and beans.
- Avoid foods high in lactose. This includes milk, ice cream, and soft cheeses. Instead have lactose-free milk, hard cheeses, yogurt, and sorbet.
- Avoid fatty, greasy, fried foods. This includes cream sauces and gravies. Limit the amount of butter and oil you use.

Taking in adequate amounts of fluids and nutrients is important for your health. If you feel that seeing a nutritionist would help you in selecting appropriate foods, ask your doctor or nurse for a referral.

> **Call your doctor or nurse if your diarrhea does not respond within 12 hours to the medications you are taking and to changes in your diet. If you have severe diarrhea and are not able to replace the fluid you lose, you can become severely dehydrated.**

58. What can I do to manage constipation?

Lisa's comment:

Constipation was probably my biggest complaint with treatment—related to my anti-nausea medications. Although intellectually I was prepared, my actual discomfort was incomprehensible. I drank fluids, I took stool softeners and laxatives, but I still had difficulty. I never had to succumb to the big guns (lactulose) but probably would have if my therapy with adriamycin/cyclophosphamide continued.

About 95% of patients with cancer have constipation at some point during the course of their treatment. This may present as infrequent bowel movements, incomplete emptying of the bowels, the passage of hard stool, or discomfort or difficulty in passing stool.

Cancer can cause constipation in a number of ways. If a tumor grows in or around the colon or rectum, it may block the passage of stool. If a tumor compresses the spinal cord, it may damage the nerves that stimulate emptying of the bowel. If a tumor causes changes in blood chemistry, there may be slowing of the movement of stool through the intestine. Cancer treatments can also cause constipation. Certain chemotherapy drugs (for example, vinblastine, vincristine, vinorelbine), antinausea medications, and pain medications can slow the movement of stool through the intestine. There are many other causes of constipation that patients with cancer may have to reckon with. These include increasing age, decreased physical activity, inadequate fiber in your diet, inadequate fluid intake, not taking the time to move your bowels, a variety of medications, and certain medical conditions like diabetes, hypothyroidism, Parkinson's disease, and depression.

If you feel you are constipated, describe your symptoms to your doctor or nurse. Tell them how often you pass your stools, the consistency of the stool, if it is painful when you have a bowel movement, and if you have any abdominal pain or cramping.

Form some regular daily routines to help train your bowel.

There is a variety of things you can do to prevent and treat constipation. First, form some regular daily routines to help train your bowel. Try to move your bowels at the same time each day. Many people feel the strongest urge right after breakfast. When you feel the urge to move your bowels, go right away; try not to hold it in. Daily exercise, especially walking, helps stimulate movement of stool within the intestines. Changes in your diet can also help with constipation. Drink six to eight glasses of fluid a day. Add fiber to your diet. Include fruit, vegetables, whole grains, and high fiber cereals.

When changes in daily routine and diet are not enough, there is a variety of medications available to help with constipation. Many of these can be purchased over the counter; however, some require a prescription. Taking a combination of a stool softener (for example, docusate) and a laxative (for example, senna, bisacodyl, lactulose, polyethylene glycol) on a regular basis can help. Ask your doctor or nurse which medications you should take, what dose, and how often you should take these.

URINARY PROBLEMS
59. What can I do for frequent urination?

Frequent urination is the need to urinate (void) more often than every 2 hours or more than eight times in a 24-hour period. If this occurs during the night, it is called **nocturia**. Some people feel like they have to void again just after they have finished going to the bathroom. Frequent urination may be accompanied by other symptoms. Urgency is the sudden sometimes uncontrollable need to urinate; this may be so strong that people leak urine before they reach the bathroom. Some people also have pain, burning, and/or a change in the color of the urine (cloudy or bloody).

Nocturia
frequent urination that occurs at night.

There are several causes of frequent urination:

- Increase in fluid intake
- Diuretics (water pills, for example, furosemide)
- Diabetes
- Urinary tract infection (UTI)
- Urinary retention (when the bladder does not fully empty all urine)
- Benign prostatic hypertrophy (BPH) (an enlargement of the prostate gland that makes it difficult for the bladder to empty)
- **Cystitis** (an inflammation or irritation of the bladder that can be caused by radiation therapy to the pelvic area, chemotherapy instilled into the bladder to treat bladder cancer, or certain chemotherapy drugs given through a vein [cyclophosphamide or ifosfamide])

Cystitis
inflammation or irritation of the bladder.

Frequent urination can interfere with your normal daily routine, causing you to stay home more than you normally would, and it can interrupt sleep, making you more tired than usual. If you have frequent urination, discuss this with your doctor or nurse. Tell them when it started, how many times you urinate during the day and night, and if you have any other symptoms in addition to the frequency. They may ask for a sample of urine to test to see if you have an infection. Other tests (for example, CT scan, ultrasound) may be performed depending on the symptoms you have and the results of the urine tests.

Most cancer patients are encouraged to drink 2 to 3 quarts of fluid per day. This by itself will cause frequent urination. To avoid waking in the night to urinate, stop drinking fluids about 3 to 4 hours before you go to sleep. If you are taking a **diuretic** (water pill), check with your doctor to see if you can take it earlier

Diuretic
a medication that increases the production of urine; also called a "water pill".

in the day to reduce the need to urinate at night. If you have diabetes and your sugar is very high, you will urinate more often. Make sure that you take your medications and check your sugar according to your doctor's instructions.

Infection is one of the most common causes of frequent urination in people with cancer. Urinary tract infections (UTIs) are usually associated with other symptoms, such as burning or pain on urination, pain in the back (flank pain), cloudy or foul smelling urine, or urine that is dark yellow or has blood in it. Sometimes people also have lower abdominal pain and a fever. If the urinalysis and urine culture show that you have an infection, the doctor will prescribe an antibiotic for you.

> **If you have symptoms of a urinary tract infection, a fever above 100.5°F, and/or shaking chills, call your doctor immediately.**

If you have an enlarged prostate gland (BPH) that is causing frequent urination or if you have urinary retention from some other cause, your doctor may prescribe medicine for you or refer you to a **urologist** (a specialist in urinary problems).

Urologist
a doctor who specializes in problems or diseases of the urinary tract.

If your urinary frequency is from treatment with radiation therapy and/or chemotherapy, the symptoms should get better with time after the treatment is completed. Your doctor may prescribe medication to help. For example, oxybutynin may be prescribed to reduce bladder spasms.

It is important that you continue to drink enough fluid during the day. Decreasing or eliminating alcohol and caffeine will also help. Keep up with your usual activities and do not stay at home all the time. Try to urinate on a set schedule. Keep a diary of when you urinate during the day and when you drink fluids to help you plan activities outside of the house and plan bathroom breaks.

For more information on urinary problems and BPH, contact the American Foundation for Urologic Diseases at *www.afud.org*.

60. What can I do for burning with urination?

Burning or pain when you urinate is called **dysuria**. It may be accompanied by other symptoms, such as frequency, urgency, and nocturia (see Question 59 for more information). If you have a vaginal infection or a rash in the area, this can cause burning when you urinate from skin irritation. Causes of dysuria include the following:

- Urinary tract infection (UTI)
- **Prostatitis** (inflammation or infection of the **prostate gland** in men)
- Cystitis (an inflammation or irritation of the bladder that can be caused by radiation therapy to the pelvic area, chemotherapy instilled into the bladder to treat bladder cancer, or certain chemotherapy drugs given through a vein [cyclophosphamide or ifosfamide])

If it is determined that you have a urinary tract infection (see Question 59) or prostatitis, your doctor will prescribe antibiotics. You should also drink at least 2 quarts of fluid each day.

Dysuria

pain or burning on urination; usually caused by irritation or infection of the bladder or urinary tract.

Prostatitis

inflammation or infection of the prostate gland.

Prostate gland

a gland within the male reproductive system that is located just below the bladder surrounding part of the urethra, the canal that empties the bladder; produces a fluid that forms part of semen.

Cyclophosphamide and ifosfamide can cause irritation of the bladder resulting in burning and sometimes blood-tinged urine. To prevent this, you will be given extra intravenous fluids with the chemotherapy and instructed to drink large amounts of fluid for 1 to 2 days after chemotherapy. You will also be asked to empty your bladder on a regular schedule. If you are getting ifosfamide, your doctor will also prescribe an intravenous medicine called Mesna that protects the lining of the bladder.

Radiation therapy to the pelvis can also cause irritation to the bladder with burning, frequency, and urgency. This can begin 3 to 5 weeks after the start of treatment and usually subsides 2 or more weeks after completion of therapy. Irritation of the bladder from chemotherapy or radiation therapy is managed in a similar way. Increase the fluid that you drink to 1 to 2 quarts every day and avoid alcohol and caffeine. If you have pain on urination, your doctor may prescribe a medicine called phenazopyridine (Pyridium). This medicine is a local analgesic that specifically works on the lining of the bladder to reduce the burning or pain. It will make your urine dark yellow or orange and it can stain your clothing.

Drink 1 to 2 quarts of fluids every day; avoid alcohol and caffeine.

> **If you have burning with urination with a fever above 100.5°F, shaking chills, flank pain, severe abdominal pain, or frank red blood or blood clots when you urinate, call your doctor.**

61. What can I do for incontinence?

Incontinence is the uncontrolled loss or leakage of urine. Anything that interferes with the muscles of the bladder or pelvic floor or the nerves in this area can

Incontinence
urinary incontinence is the uncontrolled loss or leakage of urine.

affect your ability to control urine. There are different types of incontinence. Stress incontinence is when you leak urine when you sneeze, cough, laugh, or exercise. This is usually from weakened pelvic floor muscles. Urge incontinence is when you lose urine because you cannot get to the bathroom in time. Overflow incontinence is when the amount of urine exceeds the bladder capacity, causing leakage. Or you may have no control over urination and lose large amounts of urine all the time. Incontinence, if bad enough, can keep you from enjoying your normal activities and can cause skin irritation and breakdown. Causes of incontinence include the following:

- Aging and childbirth, which can cause weakening of the pelvic floor muscles
- Urinary tract infection or inflammation
- Surgery to remove the prostate for an enlarged prostate gland (BPH) or prostate cancer
- Neurologic problems, for example metastasis (spread) of cancer to the spinal cord

If you have incontinence, describe the symptoms as clearly as you can to the doctor. He or she may order certain tests and in some cases will recommend that you see a specialist, called a urologist, a doctor who specializes in urinary problems.

> **If you are incontinent of urine and have back pain or difficulty walking or moving your bowels, call your doctor.**

Depending on the cause, incontinence may be a short-lived problem or may be permanent. Incontinence from infection or inflammation usually goes away when this resolves. Incontinence from prostate surgery, neurologic problems, childbirth, or aging can last several months or in some cases be permanent.

There are several things you can do to help with incontinence. The first is to keep a diary of when you have loss of urine. If you notice that this occurs every 2 hours, then try to urinate every hour and a half, whether you feel the need to urinate or not. If this is successful, you may be able to train your bladder and increase the length of time between visits to the bathroom. It is also important to continue to drink the amount of fluids prescribed by your doctor. To avoid incontinence at night, stop drinking fluids 4 to 5 hours before bedtime.

Ask your doctor or nurse to teach you **Kegel exercises** to strengthen your pelvic floor muscles. These are performed by squeezing (contracting) the same muscle that you use to stop urinating. If you perform this exercise regularly, you may be able to improve your ability to control your urine.

Kegel exercises
exercises designed to increase muscle strength and elasticity in the pelvis; may be recommended for treatment of urinary incontinence.

Keep your skin clean and dry. Regularly wash your genitals, groin, buttocks, and upper thigh skin with soap and water to remove any urine. Your doctor or nurse can prescribe lotion to protect the skin in this area. Additionally, pads or briefs with absorbent material can help protect your skin. Change them as soon as they become wet. If you notice redness, rash, or breakdown of skin in this area, notify your doctor or nurse.

If it is determined that your incontinence is caused by an overactive bladder muscle (detrusor muscle), your doctor may prescribe medication such as propantheline, oxybutynin, and tolterodine. These relax your bladder muscle and allow it to hold more urine, decreasing the urge to urinate. It is important that you take this medicine exactly as prescribed.

Depending on the cause, your doctor may recommend that you see a urologist, a doctor who specializes in urinary problems. The urologist may recommend a surgical procedure or teach you how to catheterize yourself. This involves inserting a thin tube through the urethra into the bladder and allowing the urine to drain. For more information on incontinence, contact the American Foundation for Urologic Diseases at *www.afud.org* or the National Association for Continence at *www.nafc.org* or 800-252-3337.

PART SIX

Appearance and Sexual Issues

I have gained weight from my cancer treatment. What can I do to lose weight?

I have developed menopause from my treatment. How can I manage the symptoms?

I am not able to get or maintain an erection since my treatment. How can this be treated?

More . . .

62. I have gained weight from my cancer treatment. What can I do to lose weight?

Most people believe that a diagnosis or treatment for cancer will cause them to lose weight. However, many people actually gain weight. This can be from the cancer, the treatment for cancer, or side effects of cancer treatment.

Some cancers cause you to accumulate large amounts of fluid, which results in weight gain. For example, cancers of the ovary, colon, or liver and metastatic cancer to the liver can cause accumulation of fluid in the abdomen, called ascites (see Question 77). Cancers or treatments for cancer that cause **lymphedema** (swelling in the arms or legs) can also cause you to gain weight (see Question 76).

If your chemotherapy treatment requires you to drink a lot of fluid or to be given large amounts of intravenous fluids, you may notice that you have gained weight after your chemotherapy treatment. This occurs in people given cisplatin or certain "high-dose" chemotherapies. Usually, your body will eliminate this fluid on its own, several days after chemotherapy.

Docetaxel is a type of chemotherapy that when given in repeated doses can commonly cause you to retain fluid. Your doctor will prescribe dexamethasone (a steroid) before and after docetaxel to prevent **fluid retention**. It is important that you take this medicine as directed.

Steroids may also be prescribed for other problems related to your cancer. Steroids can increase your appetite and can cause you to retain fluid. Thus, long-

Lymphedema

a condition in which lymph fluid collects in tissues after removal or damage to lymph nodes, from surgery or radiation therapy; usually occurs in an arm or leg.

Fluid retention

a condition in which the body does not eliminate adequate fluid and can cause swelling and weight gain.

Steroids

medications that are used to relieve swelling and inflammation; in people with cancer, steroids can be used to help other problems such as nausea and vomiting, pain, trouble breathing, and loss of energy.

term treatment with steroids (taken every day) can also cause you to gain weight. Some treatments for cancer can cause nausea or indigestion (heartburn). Very often people who have a "low level" of nausea or indigestion find that eating relieves the symptoms. There are medicines to help reduce these symptoms, reducing the need to eat increased amounts of food. See Questions 54 to 56 for more information on the treatment of heartburn and nausea.

Excessive weight gain can make it difficult to get around, cause added stress on your legs and joints, and make you short of breath. Additionally, weight gain can affect the way you feel about your appearance. If you gain weight while you are getting treatment for cancer, tell your doctor or nurse. They can help you to determine the cause of the weight gain, and they can help you to lose weight. If your weight gain is from fluid retention, your doctor may prescribe a diuretic (water pill); this will help your body eliminate the excess fluid.

If your weight gain is caused by overeating, simple measures such as eliminating second helpings, eating smaller portions, and eliminating sweets and fried foods may help you to lose weight. While you are getting treatment for cancer, it is important that you eat a well-balanced diet even if you want to lose weight. "Fad diets" and herbal weight loss products are not recommended because they may be unhealthy. Your doctor or nurse can refer you to a dietitian or nutritionist to help you with diet and weight loss.

Exercise is also important to help lose weight or prevent weight gain, and it has other benefits for people who are getting cancer treatment (see Question 34).

Appearance and Sexual Issues

121

Exercise does not need to be strenuous or complicated. Even taking a daily walk is good for you and will help you to lose or maintain your weight.

63. I have developed menopause from my treatment. How can I manage the symptoms?

Menopause is the cessation of menses (menstrual period) for a period of 12 consecutive months and results from loss of ovarian function. The ovaries produce hormones called estrogen and progesterone; when the ovaries stop making hormones, menstruation stops. All women will experience menopause, either naturally, as part of the aging process, or spontaneously, as a result of medical treatment. For most women, natural menopause occurs between the ages of 40 and 58 years. Perimenopause is a term that describes the period of time (usually between 6 to 10 years) that precedes menopause. During this time, menstrual periods may be irregular and some symptoms of menopause may be present.

Spontaneous menopause is induced by medical treatment. Surgical removal of both ovaries induces permanent menopause and immediate symptoms. Radiotherapy to the pelvis and some types of chemotherapy can cause damage to the ovaries, resulting in either temporary or permanent menopause. Symptoms may occur very soon after starting treatment or after a few months of treatment. The chemotherapy agents that most commonly cause menopause are the alkylating agents, for example, cyclophosphamide and nitrogen mustard.

Symptoms of menopause vary from person to person; they can be more intense in younger women and in women with spontaneous menopause. The most common symptoms are

- Hot flashes (or flushes) and/or night sweats;
- Sleep disturbances or insomnia;
- Anxiety;
- Decreased memory and concentration;
- Dryness, itching, and burning of the vagina and labia;
- Increase in vaginal or bladder infections;
- Decrease in sexual desire.

Additionally, the risk of **osteoporosis** (thinning of the bones) and coronary heart disease is increased during menopause.

It is important to remember that not all women will have symptoms from menopause, and if you do have symptoms, most of these will go away over time without any treatment. Until recently, hormone replacement therapy (HRT) was recommended for many women who experienced menopausal symptoms. HRT includes treatment with estrogen with or without progestin. Currently, the FDA recommends that HRT be given only for the symptoms of hot flashes, night sweats, vaginal dryness, and osteoporosis (thin weak bones). HRT is given in the lowest dose that helps your symptoms and for the shortest time that you need it. HRT is not recommended for women with some types of cancer, irregular vaginal bleeding, a history of having had a stroke or heart attack in the last year, a history of blood clots, or liver disease. Whether or not you take HRT is a decision that you and your doctor will make together.

Some women take certain complementary therapies like herbs, "natural" products, or vitamins for symp-

Osteoporosis
a condition that is characterized by a decrease in bone mass and density (thinning of the bones), causing bones to become fragile.

toms of menopause, including vitamin E, soy products, and black cohosh. At this time there is not enough information to recommend herbs or natural products for menopausal symptoms. Studies are currently being performed to determine the benefits and risks of these products. See Question 18 to learn how to get information about specific complementary therapies. Talk to your doctor or nurse before taking any medicine or herbal product (over the counter or prescription) for menopausal symptoms.

There are other measures that you can take to help you cope with menopausal symptoms. Regular exercise, such as walking or gentle aerobics, is helpful for some. Before starting any exercise program, talk to your doctor. For vaginal dryness or discomfort during sexual intercourse, vaginal moisturizers, such as Replens, and vaginal lubricants, such as Astroglide, or K-Y Jelly, may be helpful (see Question 68). Your doctor or nurse can tell you how to use these products. Ask your doctor about the use of a vaginal estrogen cream or vaginal estrogen tablets. Antianxiety or antidepressant medications are sometimes used to improve mood or decrease anxiety. Talk to your doctor about the use of these medicines. Relaxation techniques can also be helpful for reduction of stress. Your doctor or nurse can also make recommendations for the management or prevention of osteoporosis and prevention of coronary artery disease. For information on management of hot flashes, see Question 64.

For more information on menopause and management of menopausal symptoms, you can contact the North American Menopause Society at *www.menopause.org* or 440-442-7550, the National Women's Health Information Center at *www.4women.gov*, or the National Institutes of Health at *www.nhlbi.nih. gov/health/women/index.htm.*

64. *How can I manage hot flashes?*

Lisa's comment:

I was diagnosed with breast cancer at 40 years old—premenopausal. After two cycles of adriamycin/cyclophosphamide chemotherapy, over the course of one month, I experienced three unusual menstrual periods. Then the hot flashes started and my menses ended. The hot flashes intensified once I started tamoxifen therapy (post-chemotherapy). I would awaken four to five times in the night, completely soaking wet. I have been on tamoxifen for three months now and night sweats no longer awaken me. I have hot flashes throughout the day, but they are tolerable.

Hot flashes (or flushes) are the most common symptom in women during the menopausal years. They are thought to be caused by a decline in estrogen and other hormones. Other causes of hot flashes include some treatments for cancer, alcohol, caffeine, smoking, spicy food, hot showers, and hot weather. Hot flashes can also occur in men, usually as a result of hormone treatment (chemical or surgical) for prostate cancer. They can also occur as part of the normal aging process if there is a decline in the male hormone testosterone.

Hormonal therapies used for breast and prostate cancers that stop the body from producing male or female hormones or that block the activity of these hormones (see Question 7) can cause hot flashes. Usually, the frequency of the hot flashes will decrease the longer you take the medication. Radiation therapy to the pelvis and certain chemotherapy medicines given for cancer treatment can also cause a decline in hormones and cause hot flashes.

During a hot flash, you may feel warm or hot and may perspire or have "sweats." Your skin will feel warm and it may become red. Hot flashes can occur any time during the day, but most often they occur at night; this can affect the amount of sleep that you get. Hot flashes are very uncomfortable for some people and may affect your ability to function normally. If you get hot flashes, they typically last for more than 1 year and in some people they can last for as long as 5 years.

Treatments are available to help you manage hot flashes.

Treatments are available to help you manage hot flashes. Your doctor or nurse can review the options with you and help you make a decision about the right treatment for you.

Hormone replacement therapy (HRT) may be an option for some women, especially those who have debilitating hot flashes and other menopausal symptoms. For more information, see Question 63. "Topical" estrogen products or "locally" acting estrogen products (estrogen vaginal ring or tablet) are another option. These estrogen products do have side effects and should be used in the lowest possible dose and for the shortest period of time necessary.

Studies have shown that antidepressants such as fluoxetine (Prozac), venlafaxine (Effexor), and paroxetine (Paxil) have all been effective in reducing hot flashes in both men and women. Usually, the doses used to treat hot flashes are lower than the doses used to treat depression. As a result, there is a decreased chance that you could have side effects from these medicines. Gabapentin (Neurontin) is an antiseizure medicine that has reduced the frequency and severity of hot flashes in both men and women. Side effects include sleepiness and dizziness. Vitamins and herbs are also commonly used to reduce hot flashes. The most common ones are vitamin E, soy products, and black cohosh. Before using any of these products, you should speak with your doctor or nurse.

Other measures such as relaxation, exercise, and biofeedback can also be helpful. You should also dress in layers, so that if you feel a hot flash starting you can remove a layer of clothing and later can add layers as needed. For some people cotton clothing is more comfortable against the skin because it more readily absorbs perspiration than synthetic clothing. Avoid substances that trigger hot flashes, for example alcoholic beverages, hot drinks, and spicy foods.

Information available regarding management of hot flashes can be found at the National Women's Health Information Center at *www.4women.gov* or the National Institutes of Health at *www.nhlbi.nih.gov/health/women/index.htm*. Treatment information regarding men and hot flashes is limited, but some information can be obtained at the American Cancer Society at *www.cancer.org* and the Prostate Cancer Foundation at *www.prostatecancerfoundation.org*.

65. My body seems different now that I have cancer. I don't feel as attractive as I used to. What can I do to feel better about myself?

Lisa's comment:

I was never big on make-up. One of the first things my fellow nurses got excited about post-mastectomy was: "Oh, now you get to go to Look Good, Feel Better." I did attend the class, learned some cosmetic tips, and got my free bag of goodies. I pretty much didn't do anything else with the stuff.

The prospect of losing my hair was upsetting. I knew all along that I didn't want to wear a wig. I figured I would wear a baseball cap, scarf, or bandana. My hair loss occurred during the hot summer months, so the bandana was perfect. The actual hair loss was disgusting. I had cut my hair semi-short so I wouldn't have to clean up long hair. I couldn't believe how much hair kept falling off my head! Handful after handful. I enjoyed freaking out my friends. Everyone would comment on how nice my haircut looked and I would pull out a clump of hair and say "Thanks. You want some?"

I must say I never felt unattractive, I just felt I stuck out like a sore thumb. That was something I didn't expect. I suppose if I wore a wig I probably wouldn't have felt that way.

Many people feel aware of changes in their body when they have been diagnosed with cancer. There may be things you can see, like scars from surgery, drainage tubes, venous catheters, loss of hair, or a change in your weight. However, there may be nothing visible at all, just a feeling that your body is different and knowing that things inside are not the way they used to be. In addition, you may not be able to do some of the things you used to do at work or at home or for enjoyment. These things may all affect how you see yourself as a person or how attractive you feel as a man or woman.

Although there may be no way to reverse these physical changes, there are things you can do to feel better about how you look. Selecting clothes that make you feel good can make a big difference. You may want to have some favorite clothes altered to fit better if you have lost weight. Some women find that using makeup, having a manicure or pedicure, and wearing scarves helps them feel better about how they look. In addition, the American Cancer Society and the Cosmetic, Toiletry, and Fragrance Association sponsor a free program, "Look Good, Feel Better," that is dedicated to helping women being treated for cancer feel better about their appearance. They teach beauty techniques that help restore your appearance and enhance your self-image. To find out if it is available in your area, you can check on their Internet site, *www.lookgoodfeelbetter.org*, or call the American Cancer Society.

It is also helpful to think about what makes you who you are. Is it the way you look? Is it what you do? Is it what you have accomplished in the past? Is it your relationships with other people? Is it who you are as an individual, those intangible things in your mind, your heart, and your soul? While recognizing that some things have changed since your diagnosis with cancer, it is important to stay connected to those other things that make you who you are. Think about the accomplishments of your life. Plan time to be with people you enjoy. Continue to involve yourself in the things that give you intellectual satisfaction. Express your thoughts and feelings to those you trust and care for. Maintain your relatedness with whatever spirituality you feel connected to. All these things will help to remind you of who you are as a person and will enhance your feelings about yourself.

It is important to stay connected to those other things that make you who you are.

66. I don't feel the desire to be sexually intimate with my partner the way I used to. What can I do to maintain my relationship with him or her?

Physical intimacy is one aspect of a loving relationship. It gives us personal pleasure and creates a feeling of closeness to our partner. Sexual intercourse is one way of being physically intimate. However, you may find that pain, fatigue, emotional distress, or the side effects of treatment affect your desire for sex or your ability to enjoy sex.

If you would like to continue having sexual intercourse with your partner, consider strategies that will make it more pleasurable for you. Take medications that have been prescribed for any symptoms that are bothersome to you. Select a time of day when you usually have more energy and when you know you will have privacy. Experiment with different positions that might be more comfortable or less tiring. Of course, be sure to always use a safe method of birth control if there is a risk of pregnancy.

There are many other ways of maintaining a physically intimate relationship with your partner without having intercourse. Cuddling, hugging, touching, rubbing, and holding hands are some of the ways you can experience pleasure and can give pleasure. Talk with your partner about your feelings concerning your physical relationship, your fears and concerns, and your hopes and desires. Talking together about these things will create a feeling of intimacy between you and will help each of you know what the other wants and needs so that you can experience pleasure being together.

Talk with your partner about your feelings concerning your physical relationship.

Discuss your concerns with and ask questions of your doctor and nurse. They can explain how your disease and treatment may affect your sexuality. There are also sex therapists that can provide counseling to you. You can get a referral from your doctor or nurse, from the Cancer Information Service of the National Cancer Institute, or from the American Association of Sex Educators,

Counselors and Therapists at *www.aasect/org*. In addition, the American Cancer Society has two excellent books that can be helpful: *Sexuality and Cancer: For the Woman Who Has Cancer, and Her Partner* and *Sexuality and Cancer: For the Man Who Has Cancer, and His Partner*.

67. I am not able to get or maintain an erection since my treatment. How can this be treated?

Inability to get and/or maintain an erection is called erectile dysfunction. Cancer and treatment for cancer (radiation therapy and surgery) may affect erectile function. Multiple studies have shown that sexual functioning is an important aspect of quality of life for men with cancer. Sexuality and physical intimacy are ways that men and women express themselves in intimate relationships, and erectile dysfunction may interfere with this.

The sexual response in men involves four phases. First is the desire for intimacy. Second is excitement. Nerves stimulate blood vessels in the penis to dilate or open up; the increased blood flow in the penis causes it to become erect or "hard." The third phase is orgasm, the "climax" or "coming." This is the sensation of pleasure and the time when semen is pushed out of the penis, causing an ejaculation. The fourth and final phase is when blood drains out of the penis and it loses its erection.

There are many different causes of erectile dysfunction in men with cancer. It is also important to remember that this can occur as part of the normal aging process. Causes of erectile dysfunction include

- Surgery for cancer;
- Radiation therapy to the pelvis;
- Hormonal therapy for cancer;
- Symptoms from cancer or cancer treatment;
- Changes in your body that alter how you feel about yourself.

Some types of cancer surgery in the pelvis can permanently injure or require the removal of the nerve required for getting and maintaining an erection. There are now "nerve-sparing" surgeries that may increase your chances of being able to get or maintain an erection. Before having surgery for prostate, colorectal, or other cancers of the genital or urinary tract, you should speak to your surgeon about the chances of nerve injury and if it is possible to have **nerve-sparing surgery**.

Nerve-sparing surgery

a surgical procedure for men with prostate cancer in which the prostate is surgically removed and the nerves are left undisturbed with the goal of maintaining erectile function.

Radiation therapy to the pelvis may injure the blood vessels that bring blood into the penis, resulting in erectile dysfunction. Hormonal therapy for prostate cancer reduces the testosterone level, resulting in loss of desire for sex and erectile dysfunction. In addition, symptoms from cancer or cancer treatment, such as fatigue, nausea, and pain, and changes in how you feel about yourself can cause a loss of desire for sex, resulting in an inability to have an erection.

If you are having problems getting or maintaining an erection, speak to your doctor or nurse. They may want to do a blood test to check your hormone levels. The recommended treatment will depend on the results of a physical examination, blood test(s), and your prior medical and sexual history. Treatments include prescription medicine (Viagra, Levitra, Cialis), vacuum constriction devices, penile injections, and permanent penile implants. Professional counseling or sex therapy may also be helpful. Your doctor or a specialist in erectile dysfunction (urologist) will help you determine what the best option is for you.

For more information, the American Cancer Society has an excellent booklet on sexuality for men after cancer treatment. You can call 800-ACS-2345 or you can contact them on the Internet at *www.cancer.org*.

68. My doctor said there would be changes in my vagina after treatment. What does this mean and how can I treat this?

Vaginal changes can occur as a result of anything that alters a woman's production of estrogen. Estrogen is responsible for making the vagina moist and gives it the ability to elongate and become wider during sexual activity. A decrease or loss of estrogen causes vaginal dryness. In addition, the vaginal lining thins and the vaginal walls lose their ability to stretch, causing vaginal tightness. After pelvic radiation or some types of gynecologic surgery, you may develop scar tissue in the area and experience vaginal shortening and narrowing. If the tissues are not adequately stretched on a regular basis after treatment, this can cause discomfort during intercourse and make it difficult for you to be examined to determine whether there is recurrence of your cancer.

If you develop vaginal changes from your treatment, you may experience discomfort during sexual intercourse (called **dyspareunia**) or during a pelvic examination. You may also experience symptoms of vaginal dryness or irritation, which can cause discomfort during walking, sitting, or wearing pants. As a result of vaginal dryness or atrophy, you may also be more prone

Dyspareunia
pain or discomfort during sexual intercourse.

133

to vaginal yeast infections and urinary tract infections (see Question 59), and you may have vaginal bleeding from irritation during intercourse.

Before you start treatment for your cancer, speak to your doctor or nurse about the vaginal changes that can occur as a result of your treatment. Ask them to tell you ways you can minimize or prevent some of these changes.

Vaginal dryness or irritation can be helped by using vaginal moisturizers such as Replens or Senselle; these can be used every night or every other night. You should use a moisturizer even if you are not having sexual intercourse. Before sexual intercourse you may also want to use a vaginal lubricant to relieve discomfort. It is best to use a water-based, fragrance- and color-free product such as K-Y Jelly or Astroglide. Avoid oil-based products such as mineral oil or Vaseline. Some women have even found that use of a spermicidal jelly or natural yogurt relieves discomfort during intercourse. Warming the lubricants or moisturizers in warm water before use can improve comfort. Vaginal dryness or irritation can also be helped by wearing loose-fitting cotton panties and pants. Avoid using douches because these may cause further vaginal dryness and irritation.

Hormone replacement therapy or vaginal creams or rings with estrogen may also provide relief of vaginal symptoms. Hormonal medicines require a prescription, and they are not used in women with certain types of cancer. You should discuss the advantages and disadvantages of using these products with your doctor or nurse. See Question 63 for more information on hormone replacement therapy.

Vaginal discharge, burning, or itching may be signs of a vaginal infection. Some types of vaginal infections can be passed to your sexual partner during sexual activity. If you develop these symptoms, you will need to contact your doctor or nurse. They will prescribe a medication, usually a vaginal cream, to eliminate the infection. Sometimes your partner may also need to be treated with medication.

If you have had certain types of gynecologic surgery or pelvic radiation, you should stretch the vaginal walls on a regular basis to prevent narrowing and shortening. Having sexual intercourse and/or using a dilator three times a week can accomplish this. Vaginal dilators are easy to use. Your doctor or nurse will give you instructions on how to use a vaginal dilator, and they will tell you how long you should wait after radiotherapy or surgery before using it.

For more information the American Cancer Society has an excellent booklet on women's sexuality after cancer treatment. You can call 800-ACS-2345 or you can contact them on the Internet at *www.cancer.org*.

69. Will I be able to conceive a child after treatment?

Lisa's comment:

I never felt that I wanted to have children. This decision and reality was acceptable because I was not married. At forty and single, being diagnosed with breast cancer and having to undergo chemotherapy and then tamoxifen therapy, I was faced with the permanence of my pre-breast cancer reality. I would never have children. I was surprised by my sudden concern and inner turmoil about being childless. Having the choice taken away from me was very upsetting, and I still get emotional thinking about it.

For many people, the ability to have children is one of the most important aspects of their lives. This may be a major concern for those who are getting treatment for cancer and for their families. For some people, reproductive ability is permanently affected by cancer or treatment for cancer; in others, the ability to have a child will return when their cancer treatment is completed. Other concerns regarding fertility or pregnancy after cancer treatment include the ability to carry a child to term and the ability to deliver a healthy baby.

The ability to conceive a child is a complicated process that depends on the production of healthy sperm, healthy eggs, and the general health of the woman's reproductive organs. Reproductive problems can affect both men and women and can be caused by cancer, cancer treatment that affects sexual organs or sexual hormones, or the natural aging process. Surgery for testicular, prostate, or penile cancer may affect a man's ability to have children, whereas surgery for ovarian, uterine, cervical, or vaginal cancer may cause a woman to become unable to have a child. Some types of chemotherapy, hormone therapy, and radiation therapy to the pelvis can also temporarily or permanently affect fertility. There are other factors or medical conditions that can also affect fertility in men and women:

Reproductive problems can affect both men and women.

- **Endometriosis** (a problem related to the lining of the uterus)
- Infections such as prostatitis or pelvic inflammatory disease
- Low sperm count
- Sexually transmitted diseases

Endometriosis
a benign condition in which tissue similar to that which lines the uterus grows in abnormal places in the abdomen.

If you have cancer and you are in your reproductive years, speak to your doctor or nurse before undergoing any treatment for cancer. Many options are available for both men and women to help them conceive a child after treatment for cancer, such as sperm banking, in vitro fertilization, donor eggs, and the use of surrogate mothers. If these options are not possible, you may want to consider adoption.

Sperm banking is an option for men and, if desired, should be done before any cancer treatment begins. Ask your doctor or nurse to give you the name of a sperm bank in your area. Sperm banking can be done in 1 day and therefore should not cause any delay in treatment for cancer. This procedure involves production of a sample of sperm; this is usually accomplished by masturbation and then ejaculation of sperm into a special container. After production of the sample, the sperm is analyzed and then frozen (cryopreserved). After treatment, if you want to start a family, the sperm is thawed and then used to inseminate your partner. Sperm banking is not usually covered by insurance; however, it is affordable for most people.

Egg harvesting for in vitro fertilization (IVF) may be an option for some women. IVF is a procedure that involves the surgical removal (harvesting) of a woman's eggs from her ovaries. To produce an adequate number of eggs, women are given hormones for several weeks. Just before ovulation is anticipated, the eggs are harvested. After the eggs are removed, they are mixed with sperm outside the body in a Petri dish. After about one and a half days, the eggs are examined to see whether they have become fertilized by the sperm. Any fertilized eggs (embryos) can then be frozen. When a woman wants to conceive a child, the embryos are thawed and then implanted into her uterus. Alternatively, if you are not able to carry a child, the embryo can be implanted in the uterus of a

Many options are available for both men and women to help them conceive a child after treatment for cancer.

Appearance and Sexual Issues

surrogate mother. IVF is a long and complicated process and would require a delay in the start of cancer treatment. IVF is partly covered by most insurance companies; however, it is still an expensive process.

IVF and egg-harvesting procedures are called assisted reproductive technologies. The same techniques that are used to harvest eggs for IVF can also be used to obtain donor eggs from another woman if you are infertile. These donor eggs are fertilized by your partner's sperm, producing embryos, and can be implanted in your uterus or in the uterus of a surrogate mother.

The decision that you and your partner make regarding having a family is a very personal one. It is important to remember that there is not one right decision. Some people may decide to use the reproductive technologies that are available to them, some may decide not to have children, and still others may decide to adopt children. Facing treatment for cancer is difficult, and concerns about the ability to have a family can cause added stress.

To locate sperm banks in your area, go to *www. spermbankdirectory.com*. For more information regarding sperm banking, IVF, and other reproductive technologies in patients who are undergoing treatment for cancer, you can contact the following:

- American Cancer Society at *www.cancer.org* 800-ACS-2345
- National Cancer Institute at *www.cancer.gov* or 800-4-CANCER
- American Society for Reproductive Medicine at *www.asrm.org*
- Surrogacy, Embryo and Egg Donor Services at *www.seedscenter.com* or 800-733-1673

PART SEVEN

Neurologic Problems, Fluid Retention, and Blood Chemistry

What is peripheral neuropathy
and how is this managed?

What is cerebral edema? How is this managed?

Why are my legs swollen?
What can I do to minimize this?

What is a pleural effusion? How is this treated?

How is treatment-related
diabetes diagnosed and treated?

More . . .

NEUROLOGIC PROBLEMS AND INFLAMMATION

70. What is peripheral neuropathy and how is this managed?

Lisa's comment:

My experience with peripheral neuropathy was surprising. As an oncology nurse (16 years) I have taught the signs and symptoms of chemotherapy toxicities thousands of times. So, you would think I'd recognize a symptom. With my first paclitaxel treatment I noticed that my hands and wrists were itchy about three days after therapy. I would be at work and I'd go crazy scratching. I was out to lunch with a co-worker one afternoon and started complaining about my weird itching sensations localized to the wrists/hands, and she said: "You're having peripheral neuropathies." I was shocked. Over the years, I'd never heard one patient complain of pruritis in the "glove" area only. By my last paclitaxel cycle, the classic numbness and tingling presented itself in both my hands and feet. However, the symptoms improved a few weeks off treatment.

Peripheral neuropathy

a condition of the nervous system that causes numbness, tingling, burning or weakness; usually begins in the hands or feet and can be caused by certain anticancer drugs.

Peripheral neuropathy is a term that describes damage to peripheral nerves. The peripheral nerves are the nerves outside the brain and spinal cord. There are three types of peripheral nerves: sensory, motor, and autonomic. Sensory nerves allow us to feel temperature, pain, vibration, and touch. Motor nerves are responsible for voluntary movement; they allow us to walk and open doors, for example. Autonomic nerves control involuntary or automatic functions such as breathing, digestion, sweating, and bowel and bladder function. When there is damage to the peripheral nerves, the symptoms that occur depend on which peripheral nerves are affected.

Peripheral neuropathy can occur in people with diabetes, alcoholism, and with severe malnutrition. Some antibiotics (for example, ciprofloxacin, levofloxacin) can cause peripheral neuropathy. In people who have cancer, the most common cause of peripheral neuropathy is chemotherapy. Chemotherapy can affect any of the peripheral nerves but most commonly affects the sensory nerves, causing numbness and tingling in the hands and feet. The following chemotherapy medicines can cause damage to peripheral nerves: paclitaxel, cisplatin, carboplatin, oxaliplatin, vincristine, vinorelbine, and thalidomide. If you have peripheral neuropathy from another cause, chemotherapy can sometimes make it worse.

In people who have cancer, the most common cause of peripheral neuropathy is chemotherapy.

Symptoms of peripheral neuropathy include

- Numbness and tingling ("pins and needles") in hands and/or feet;
- Burning pain in hands and feet;
- Difficulty writing or buttoning a shirt;
- Difficulty holding a cup or glass;
- Constipation;
- Decreased sensation of hot and cold;
- Muscle weakness;
- Decreased hearing or ringing in the ears (tinnitus).

Oxaliplatin causes a unique symptom from peripheral neuropathy in almost half of all patients who receive the drug. It is an acute sensitivity to cold that starts from hours to 1 to 2 days after treatment and can last up to 14 days. If you are on oxaliplatin, do not suck on ice chips or drink cold fluids and use a straw when drinking. Do not take anything from the freezer or touch cold metal objects unless you have gloves on. Cover your mouth, nose, and head with a scarf when going outdoors in cold weather.

It is difficult to prevent chemotherapy-induced neuropathy, but if you get it, it is possible to prevent it from getting worse. If you have any of the symptoms listed above before you start chemotherapy or if you develop these symptoms while on chemotherapy, tell your doctor or nurse. Describe the symptom, tell them when it started, and if the symptom makes it harder or prevents you from performing any activities like writing a check, buttoning your shirt, or walking. Because chemotherapy can sometimes cause permanent neuropathy, be sure to talk about this before your treatment.

Most often the diagnosis of peripheral neuropathy is based on a description of the symptoms that you are having and on a physical examination. Blood tests cannot diagnose peripheral neuropathy. Sometimes your doctor may ask you to see a **neurologist** to help with diagnosis and treatment. Usually other tests are not needed.

Neurologist

a physician who takes care of people who have problems or diseases of the nervous system.

If you have neuropathy and it is interfering with your activity or causing pain, your doctor may decide to reduce the dose of chemotherapy or stop it altogether. By doing this, the neuropathy should not get worse and may even go away. Neuropathy can take from 6 to 12 months to get better or resolve completely.

Your doctor may also prescribe medication for you to take. The medicines most commonly prescribed are also used to treat seizures and depression and include gabapentin (Neurontin), carbamazepine (Tegretol), and amitriptyline (Elavil). Amitriptyline makes people sleepy, and it should be taken at bedtime. If there is pain associated with your neuropathy, your doctor may prescribe an opioid (see Question 25 on pain medicine).

If you have peripheral neuropathy, there are several safety hints that you can use at home so you don't hurt yourself. If you have numbness and tingling in your feet and have trouble walking or trip often, keep your home well lighted, avoid scatter rugs, and watch the placement of your feet when you walk. Use handrails when walking on stairs. If you drive a car, make sure you can feel the pedals with your feet. If you have trouble feeling temperature, ask someone else to test the temperature of drinks or bath water for you so you don't burn yourself. Your doctor or nurse may refer you to a physical or occupational therapist to help you to regain function.

For more information on peripheral neuropathy in people with cancer, refer to The Neuropathy Association at *neuropathy.org* and to Oncolink at *oncolink.org*.

71. What is cerebral edema? How is this managed?

Cerebral edema (or swelling of the brain) is the result of inflammation in the brain. There are many different causes of cerebral edema; two causes are stroke and head injury. In patients with cancer, the most common causes are primary brain tumors (tumors that start in the brain) or metastatic brain tumors (tumors that start elsewhere and spread to the brain). Carcinomatous meningitis can also cause cerebral edema. This is a condition caused by cancer cells that "seed" or start growing on the lining of the brain. Swelling from radi-

Cerebral edema
swelling of the brain from inflammation or other diseases.

143

ation therapy or surgery to the brain may also cause cerebral edema.

The brain is part of the central nervous system and is protected by the skull. If there is swelling in the brain, pressure can develop because the skull does not expand. This can result in neurologic symptoms. If the pressure is severe, it is called increased intracranial pressure. Symptoms of cerebral edema include the following:

• Headache
• Nausea and vomiting
• Blurred or double vision
• Difficulty walking
• Seizures
• Difficulty speaking or finding the right words
• Weakness of an extremity or one side of the body
• Personality changes or difficulty thinking

MRI is the best test to determine whether you have cerebral edema.

If you have any of these symptoms, contact your doctor or nurse. If there is concern that you have cerebral edema, they will perform a history and physical examination. They will also perform blood tests and an MRI of the head. MRI is the best test to determine whether you have cerebral edema. If you are claustrophobic or have difficulty taking an MRI, alert your health care providers; they may be able to prescribe medicine to help with this. A CT scan of the head may also be needed to determine whether you have another cause for your symptoms.

If you have cerebral edema, treatment will depend on the cause. The goal of treatment is to maintain or restore neurologic function. In nearly every case, steroid medicines are used to decrease inflammation and edema (see Question 72 for more information on steroids). If you have symptoms, they will often improve or resolve once you start steroids. If you have a seizure as a result of cerebral edema, antiseizure medicines will be prescribed. **If these medicines are given to you, it is important that you take them exactly as your doctor prescribed.** In cases of severe edema, special intravenous fluids and surgery are sometimes used to decrease edema. This requires a stay in the hospital.

If you have a primary brain tumor or a tumor that has metastasized to the brain, surgery, radiotherapy, or both are needed. Chemotherapy that goes directly to the brain (regional chemotherapy) is sometimes used to treat carcinomatous meningitis. The chemotherapy is given into an artery or into the cerebrospinal fluid that surrounds the brain.

72. What are steroids? Why are they used?

Steroids are very potent antiinflammatory medicines that doctors use for a variety of medical problems. Doctors also use steroids for many different reasons in patients who have cancer and in patients who are getting treatment for cancer. In patients who have cerebral edema from cancer, steroids are used to decrease the swelling in the brain and to reduce neurologic symptoms caused by the swelling. Steroids have also been found to be helpful in preventing nausea and vomiting from chemotherapy. Steroids are usually given in pill form, although sometimes they are given intravenously (by vein). The steroid that is most often used in these situations is dexamethasone. Other steroid medicines that are sometimes used are hydrocortisone, methylprednisolone, and prednisone.

Before you start to take steroids, talk to your doctor or nurse about the potential side effects and how to take the medicine. Side effects are more common if you are taking this medicine for a longer period of time. These side effects are as follows:

- Muscle weakness
- Weight gain
- Difficulty sleeping
- Increased blood sugar
- Indigestion or stomach ulcer
- Osteoporosis
- Personality changes
- Increased risk for infection

Some of these side effects can be prevented or minimized. To avoid stomach upset or ulcer, always take your steroid medicine with food. Your doctor may also prescribe an antiulcer pill for you to take (for example, omeprazole or lansoprazole). If you have difficulty sleeping, ask if you can take the medicine early in the day. If you have diabetes, steroid use may increase your blood sugar. Because of this your doctor may want to monitor your blood sugar more closely, or he or she may recommend some changes in your diabetes medicines. If you are at risk for osteoporosis, your doctor will prescribe calcium and/or a medicine like alendronate (Fosamax) or pamidronate, which strengthens the bones. If you are at risk for infection, your doctor may give you a special antibiotic to prevent this.

If you are taking the steroid medicine for 2 or more weeks, your doctor will taper you slowly off the medicine. This means that he or she will reduce the total daily dose slowly over several days to weeks.

> **It is very important that you take the steroid medicine exactly as your doctor prescribes and that you do not stop taking the medicine abruptly.**

73. I am having trouble remembering things and feel confused at times. What can I do about this?

People with cancer or people who are getting treatment for cancer sometimes have trouble remembering names, places, or events or have trouble with language skills, concentration, or arithmetic. This problem is called **cognitive dysfunction**. Scientists are now studying this problem in patients with cancer, and they have found that some degree of impairment is common. Although most of the time the impairment is subtle, it can still be quite bothersome to patients.

Cognitive dysfunction

difficulty remembering names, places, or events or trouble with language skills, concentration, or arithmetic.

Lisa's comment:

My friends and I would joke about it—"Oh, it's that chemo brain again!" I would forget things they'd tell me or have difficulty verbalizing myself. It was quite frustrating at times, but a good excuse at other times! I definitely see improvement in my cognitive function now that I am off chemotherapy.

Paraneoplastic syndrome

a group of symptoms that may develop when substances released by some cancer cells disrupt the normal function of cells and tissue away from the tumor; it can be a cause of cognitive dysfunction.

There are many causes of cognitive impairment. It may be a direct effect of a tumor in the brain (for example, cerebral edema, metastatic brain tumor) or a remote effect of a tumor outside the brain (for example, **paraneoplastic syndrome**; see Question 81). Treatment for cancer, including chemotherapy, biologic therapy, and radiation therapy, are responsible for cognitive dysfunction in one third to one half of patients reporting

147

symptoms. Abnormal blood chemistry, certain medications, fatigue, anxiety, depression, stress, and pain can also contribute to impairment.

Treatment of cognitive dysfunction begins with finding the cause of the problem. If you experience any of the symptoms listed above, call your doctor or nurse. They will take a history and perform a physical examination. Blood tests can determine whether the problem is from abnormal blood chemistry. For example, high calcium levels in the blood can cause cognitive impairment. When this is corrected, the problem will resolve. If your difficulty stems from anxiety, depression, or pain, medicines may be prescribed to help this. If it is suspected that one of your medications, for example, a pain medicine or antibiotic, is causing the problem, your doctor may change your medication. If the problem is from fatigue and anemia, erythropoietin may be prescribed to treat the anemia (see Question 38).

If it is determined that your problem is from your cancer, treatment of the cancer may relieve the problem. If it is determined that your problem is from your treatment for cancer, there are other interventions that your doctor or nurse can prescribe. Medication is sometimes used. Donepezil hydrochloride (Aricept), a medicine used in Alzheimer's disease, has been found to be helpful in patients with cognitive impairment. Methylphenidate (Ritalin) has also been used with some success. If your symptoms are troublesome to you, discuss the possibility of having physical, vocational, or occupational therapy and cognitive rehabilitation with your doctor. These interventions have been helpful for others and may be beneficial for you by improving your daily level of functioning. In addition, many health care professionals and cancer patients have cited the benefits of daily physical and mental activity in helping with cognitive function. For more information on cognitive dysfunction and helpful interventions, consult *www.cancersymptoms.org.*

FLUID, BLOOD CHEMISTRY, AND BLOOD VESSELS

74. Why are my legs swollen? What can I do to minimize this?

There are several reasons people with cancer can develop swelling in their legs. First, when you have lost a lot of weight the amount of protein in the blood decreases, causing fluid to leak out of the blood vessels and accumulate in the tissues. The fluid accumulates in the feet, ankles, and legs because gravity pulls the fluid downward. Second, certain chemotherapy drugs and other medications may cause fluid retention. This excess fluid may leak out of the blood vessels and lead to swelling. Third, a tumor in the abdomen or pelvis can put pressure on the lymph vessels and veins coming up from the legs. These vessels run throughout your body and carry fluid that normally collects in the tissues back into the bloodstream. If the vessels become blocked, they lose their ability to carry this fluid out of the tissues, leading to swelling. Finally, blood clots (called **thrombosis**) may form in the veins of the leg, blocking the flow of blood up from the legs. This usually occurs in only one leg, so the swelling will usually be seen in only one leg. This is accompanied by inflammation of the vein, usually causing redness, heat, and/or pain in the leg as well. This condition is known as deep vein thrombosis (DVT). Patients with cancer are particularly at risk for this problem, which must be treated medically as soon as possible to prevent serious complications (see Question 75).

Thrombosis

the formation or presence of a blood clot inside a blood vessel.

Depending on the cause of swelling, a number of strategies may help reduce the swelling and improve your comfort. Be sure your shoes, socks, and pants are not too tight. This may constrict the vessels in your leg and increase the swelling. You may need to purchase shoes and socks that are bigger than your usual size. If you do not have a blood clot in your leg, you can also purchase special compression stockings at your drug store. These may improve the ability of the vessels to return excess fluid from the legs. However, it is important that these fit correctly to avoid constriction and worsening of the problem. If you notice indented rings in the skin of your legs when you remove your socks or stockings, they are too tight. Walking may also be helpful. Walking causes contractions of your leg muscles, which supports the ability of the vessels to return excess fluid from the legs. Try to walk short distances frequently throughout the day; however, avoid standing in place for long periods of time. Whenever sitting, keep your legs elevated. Position them so that your feet are higher than your knees, which are higher than your hips. This way gravity will help pull the fluid out of your legs. Water pills or diuretics may be helpful if the swelling is from fluid retention. However, some people may become dehydrated from diuretics, so they should only be taken if prescribed by your doctor. If the swelling is from fluid retention, reducing the amount of salt in your food may also be helpful.

75. What is deep vein thrombosis (DVT)? How is it diagnosed and treated?

Patients with cancer are at risk for developing deep vein thrombosis (DVT). A blood clot (called thrombosis) forms in the vein of a leg, blocking the flow of blood up from the leg which results in swelling. This is accompanied by inflammation of the vein, usually causing redness, heat, and/or pain in the leg as well. If left untreated, the blood clot will build up over time. There is the possibility that pieces of the blood clot will break off (called **emboli**) and travel to other parts of the body. These can then block a blood vessel to one of your vital organs, like the lung (called pulmonary embolus).

Emboli

blood clots that travel through blood vessels and eventually obstruct or block the flow of blood.

> **Call your doctor immediately if you develop sudden swelling in one leg with or without redness or tenderness of the calf.**

If your doctor suspects that the swelling may be from a blood clot, an ultrasound examination (**Doppler**) of your leg may be ordered. This is a simple test that visualizes the veins in your legs and detects clots that may be present.

Doppler ultrasound

a procedure in which high-energy sound waves (ultrasound) are bounced off internal tissues or organs and make echoes that form a picture of body tissues called a sonogram; used to determine if there is a blood clot in a blood vessel in an arm or leg.

If the diagnosis is confirmed, treatment with anticoagulants will be started immediately to prevent the blood from forming additional clots. Over time, the body will naturally break down the clot that has already developed. Heparin is the drug most commonly used initially. It can be given by continuous intravenous infusion, requiring hospitalization for a number of days, or by injection under the skin with a small needle several times a day. New low molecular weight heparin is increasingly being used. It provides several advantages: It can be given safely at home with only one or two injections a day, the dose can be determined more accurately than with other forms of heparin, and there is no need to have frequent blood tests to monitor its effects.

For most patients, an oral anticoagulant medication, warfarin, is also begun within a day or two of starting

151

heparin. However, warfarin takes several days to a week to reach the right level in your blood. There is no standard dose of warfarin; the dose you take will be determined by its effect on your blood. Two blood tests, the prothrombin time (PT) and the Internationalized Normal Ratio (INR), are used. Your doctor will adjust your dose of warfarin until the INR reaches a therapeutic level (between 2 and 3). At that time, the heparin is usually stopped. You will continue on the warfarin for at least 6 months; you may have to stay on this medication for the rest of your life. Throughout that time you will have to have periodic blood tests taken, anywhere from twice a week to once a month, to confirm that your dose is correct. Adjustments in the dose are made as needed to keep the INR between 2 and 3.

It is important that you take the exact dose of warfarin prescribed each night because small changes in the dose can have very large effects on your blood. If you do not take enough warfarin, there is a chance you can develop more blood clots. If you take too much, there is a chance you can develop bleeding. If you notice any signs of bleeding, contact your doctor or nurse immediately.

The metabolism of warfarin may be affected by certain foods, causing the warfarin to have either a greater or lesser effect at the same dose. Ask your pharmacist to give you a list of foods that interact with warfarin and try to avoid these while you are on this medication. In addition, warfarin can interact with a variety of medications. Always make sure to tell any doctor who prescribes medication for you that you are taking this drug.

Occasionally, patients develop new or worsening blood clots despite being treated with an adequate dose of warfarin. In this circumstance, your doctor may choose to put you back on heparin on a long-term basis. An alternative treatment would be to put a special filter, called an **inferior vena cava (IVC) filter**, in one of the large veins of your body to prevent blood clots from traveling to the lung.

76. What is lymphedema? How can I manage this?

Lymph is a fluid of water and proteins that brings nutrients to the tissues and then is absorbed into the lymphatic system, a connection of vessels and lymph nodes that carry the fluid back to the blood stream. Lymph nodes are little bean-shaped structures located under the arms, in the neck, and in the groin that filter bacteria and waste products from the lymph. A backup or blockage in this system that prevents lymph from returning to the circulatory system can cause swelling (edema) in an arm or leg. Lymph nodes and vessels are also located deep within the body, but these are not associated with lymphedema.

Inferior vena cava filter

the inferior vena cava is a large vein that empties into the heart and carries blood from the legs and feet and from organs in the abdomen and pelvis; a filter (umbrella-like device) may be placed in the inferior vena cava to prevent blood clots in the legs from traveling to the lungs.

Lymphedema is an abnormal accumulation of lymph fluid caused either by overproduction of lymph (primary lymphedema) or obstruction of the lymph vessels or nodes, causing a backup or accumulation of lymph in the tissues beneath the skin (secondary lymphedema). Lymphedema can occur anywhere in the body where lymph nodes or lymph vessels are present, but it most commonly occurs in an extremity (arm or leg), causing it to become swollen. Secondary lymphedema is the most common type in people with cancer. It is most commonly seen in people who have had removal of lymph nodes as part of their cancer treatment or who have had injury or scarring of the lymph nodes. Lymphedema can cause discomfort or

Preventive measures, early recognition, and treatment are helpful in the management of lymphedema.

pain, limitations in the use of the swollen extremity, and changes in the appearance of your body. Preventive measures, early recognition, and treatment are helpful in the management of lymphedema.

Risk factors for developing lymphedema include the following:

- Surgical removal of lymph nodes or vessels in the underarm or groin areas for treatment and staging of cancer
- Scar tissue development after surgery or radiation therapy to the underarm or groin
- Obstruction from tumor
- Cellulitis (infection) in the affected extremity
- Obesity

The incidence of lymphedema is lower in the last decade because of improvements in surgical and radiation therapy techniques. After surgery, there may be acute lymphedema, but this usually resolves once the body compensates (heals itself). Chronic lymphedema can occur from months to years after treatment for cancer. If you have lymphedema, you may experience heaviness, throbbing pain or soreness, and a feeling of tightness from your wristwatch, ring, shoes, or clothes in the affected arm or leg. In addition, your skin may become shiny and tight or brownish in color, and it may feel firm. There are other causes of swelling in an arm or leg, including development of a blood clot in a blood vessel (see Question 75) and infection.

> **Call your doctor or nurse for any new development of swelling in your arm or leg. Tell them if you also have any pain, redness, red streaks, fever (>100.5°F), chills, or shortness of breath.**

Your doctor will want to perform a physical examination and will measure the swollen extremity and compare it with your normal one. He or she may also perform other tests, such as ultrasound, CT scan, or MRI, which will tell him or her if the obstruction is in a blood vessel or lymph vessel.

If you have had surgery to remove lymph nodes as part of your cancer treatment, ask your nurse about ways to prevent lymphedema. Some prevention strategies include the following:

- Perform gentle strengthening and stretching exercises to keep the affected limb working normally.
- Avoid lifting or moving heavy objects on the side of surgery.
- Keep skin clean and moisturized, avoid cuts or cracks in the skin, and avoid insect bites.
- Avoid blood draws, intravenous lines, and blood pressure measurement in the affected arm.
- Report signs of infection to your doctor or nurse (redness, tenderness, swelling fever).
- Report other changes in your limb, including pain, numbness, or changes in skin color.

If you develop lymphedema, there are several treatments that may be helpful to you. Unfortunately, there are no medicines that are routinely used to prevent or treat lymphedema. Treatments include elevation of the affected limb, use of a compression garment such as a sleeve or stocking, massage, compression bandaging, and a pressure pump. It may also be a good idea to see a lymphedema specialist. Lymphedema specialists are usually physical therapists that have additional training in the management of lymphedema. If you have pain or are distressed as a result of your lymphedema, discuss this with your doctor; he or she can prescribe an antidepressant or pain medicine.

For more information on lymphedema, contact The National Lymphedema Network at 800-541-3259 or on the Internet at *www.lymphnet.org*. An Internet resource for people with lymphedema from treatment for breast cancer is *www.breastcancer.org*.

77. What is ascites? How is this treated?

Peritoneal cavity

the space within the abdomen that contains the intestines, stomach, and the liver; lined by thin membranes.

Ascites is an abnormal buildup of fluid in the **peritoneal cavity**. The peritoneum is a membrane that lines the abdominal cavity; one layer surrounds the abdominal and pelvic organs, whereas the other layer lines the wall of the abdominal cavity. Normally, there is a small amount of fluid in this cavity that prevents friction during organ movement. In healthy people, this fluid moves constantly in and out of the peritoneal space. In some people the cancer causes increases in the amount of fluid moving into the space or obstruction of the circulatory and lymphatic systems, causing fluid to back up, unable to move out of the space. These problems can cause accumulation of fluid in the peritoneal cavity, called malignant ascites. Cancers that can cause malignant ascites are gynecologic tumors (for example, ovary, uterus), gastrointestinal tumors (for example, colon, stomach), liver cancer, breast cancer, mesothelioma, and lymphoma. Diagnosis of ascites is accomplished by physical examination and radiologic tests, including ultrasound, CT, and/or MRI of the abdomen.

Symptoms of ascites can vary and depend on the amount of fluid in the abdomen; small amounts of fluid may cause vague symptoms, whereas larger amounts of fluid can cause more discomfort and swelling of the abdomen. If you have ascites, you may feel some of the following symptoms:

- Weight gain, with clothing fitting more tightly across the abdomen
- Abdominal bloating, discomfort, or pain
- Decreased appetite
- Indigestion
- Nausea or vomiting
- Shortness of breath
- Fatigue

If you have ascites and you have these symptoms, there are things you can do to make yourself more comfortable. If your abdomen is swollen from too much fluid, wear loose clothing. For a decreased appetite, try to eat six small meals each day, instead of two or three. Eat foods that are high in protein and calories. If you have nausea or vomiting, take antinausea medicines on a regular basis and before meals (see Question 56).

> **Call your doctor or nurse if you have ascites and you are short of breath, have uncontrolled nausea or vomiting or uncontrolled pain, or you are suddenly unable to fit into your clothes.**

In addition to the above comfort measures, your doctor may recommend removal of fluid from your abdomen. This can be accomplished by inserting a thin tube into the peritoneal space where the fluid is located. This is done with the help of an ultrasound machine. Once the tube is in the right place to drain fluid, it is attached to a drainage bag to collect the fluid. When the fluid is finished draining, the tube will be removed

Your doctor may recommend removal of fluid from your abdomen.

Paracentesis

a procedure in which a thin needle or tube is placed through the abdominal wall to the peritoneal cavity.

and the fluid discarded. This procedure is called a **paracentesis**. Usually, after paracentesis your symptoms will improve. Unfortunately, the fluid usually reaccumulates in days to weeks after paracentesis. Paracentesis can usually be performed as needed to help relieve your symptoms. For some patients, special tubes can be left in place for a period of time to allow for continual drainage of the fluid if needed.

Shunt

implantation or creation of a permanent tube to move blood or other fluid from one part of the body to another part; for example, to control ascites, sometimes a shunt is placed in the abdomen to direct the fluid into the bloodstream.

Another way to remove fluid from your abdomen involves placement of a **shunt**. This is a permanent tube placed in your abdomen that directs the fluid into your bloodstream. Once in the bloodstream, your kidneys will remove the fluid and you will eliminate it with your urine. Your doctor will recommend this procedure if it is right for you.

Sometimes, giving chemotherapy directly into the peritoneal cavity can also help to control ascites.

78. What is a pleural effusion? How is this treated?

Pleural space

the space between the membranes that line the inside of the chest wall and cover the outside of the lungs.

Pleural effusion is an abnormal buildup of fluid in the **pleural space**. The pleura are membranes that line the inside of the chest wall and cover the outside of the lungs. The space between the membranes is called the pleural space. Normally, there is a small amount of fluid in this space. This fluid provides lubrication for the lungs to expand and contract during breathing. Pleural fluid moves in and out of the pleural space. If you have fluid that builds up in this space, the lungs cannot expand normally when you inhale, causing you to have shortness of breath. Pleural effusions can occur in one or both lungs.

Pleural effusions can be caused by

- Infection (for example, pneumonia);
- Congestive heart failure;
- Surgery in the chest or abdomen;
- Cancer.

If the fluid is caused by cancer, this is called a malignant pleural effusion. Most often, cancer cells cause a buildup of fluid either by lodging in the pleura or by being present in the pleural fluid; this causes the pleura to become irritated. When this happens, extra fluid can collect in the pleural space. The cancers that most often cause pleural effusions are lung, breast, adenocarcinoma of unknown primary, mesothelioma, lymphoma, and leukemia.

Not everyone has symptoms from a pleural effusion. If the fluid collection is small, you may not have any symptoms. If there is a large amount of fluid buildup, you may experience the following symptoms:

- Fullness or heaviness in the chest
- Discomfort or pain in the chest
- Cough
- Shortness of breath

If you have these symptoms, discuss them with your doctor or nurse. Diagnosis of a pleural effusion is made by physical examination and chest x-ray. First, you will have a standing chest x-ray, and then you will be asked to lie down on your side (the side with the fluid will be down on the x-ray table) and another x-ray will be taken in this position. This is called a lateral decubitus x-ray. Pleural fluid can also be seen on a CT scan.

Treatment for pleural effusion depends on the amount of fluid in your chest and if you are having symptoms from the fluid. If you have a small or medium pleural effusion that is not causing any symptoms, your doctor may recommend chemotherapy that will treat the tumor and make the fluid go away. If you have a large pleural effusion and have shortness of breath or pain, the doctor can remove the fluid. This is done by inserting a needle through the ribs into the pleural space and removing the fluid. This is called a **thoracentesis**. You do not need to be admitted to the hospital for this procedure. If the fluid comes back, your doctor may recommend a procedure called **pleurodesis**. This is done by inserting a chest tube through the ribs into the pleural space and draining it dry. Once the fluid is removed, your doctor will insert a special medicine through the chest tube into the pleural space. This medicine causes irritation of the pleura and scar tissue to form. Once this happens, the pleura stick together, leaving no space for fluid to accumulate; for most people this permanently prevents fluid from building up again in the pleural space. This procedure is done while you are in the hospital.

Thoracentesis

removal of fluid from the pleural cavity through a needle inserted between the ribs.

Pleurodesis

a medical procedure that uses chemicals or drugs to cause inflammation and adhesion between the layers of the pleura (the tissue that covers the lungs and lines the interior wall of the chest cavity) to prevent the buildup of fluid in the pleural cavity; used as a treatment for severe pleural effusion.

If you have symptoms from a pleural effusion, there are several things you can do to make yourself more comfortable. If you have shortness of breath or breathing is difficult, your doctor may prescribe oxygen and medicine for you to make breathing easier. Sleeping on pillows or in a recliner may make breathing easier (see Question 46 for more information on management of shortness of breath). If you have pain, take your pain medicine as your doctor recommends.

79. My doctor has told me my blood chemistry can be affected by treatment. What does this mean?

A number of tests analyze the different chemicals in your blood. Blood chemistry tests include measurement of **lipids, glucose** (sugar), **electrolytes**, enzymes, vitamins, and hormones. Certain blood chemistry tests can tell us how well your different organs function. For example, liver function studies tell us how well your liver is working. Other studies tell us how well your kidneys, heart, and lungs are working. This is similar to a complete blood count (CBC), which tells us how well your bone marrow (organ which makes different blood cells) is working (see Question 35 for more information on blood counts).

Certain drugs used for cancer treatments depend on specific organs, such as the liver or kidneys, to be eliminated from the body. If these organs do not function normally, the drug levels can build up in your body and cause serious side effects.

Some treatments have the potential to damage specific organs in your body. Your doctor and nurse will do everything they can to prevent this from happening. For certain treatments they will give you large amounts of fluid intravenously or give you certain medicines before or after treatment to prevent organ damage. They may instruct you to increase the amount of fluid you drink before or after treatment. It is important that you take your medicine and drink fluid exactly as your doctor prescribes. They may even ask you to measure the amount of fluid that you drink and measure the amount of urine that you put out every day. If you are getting any treatment that can damage your organs, your doctor will

Lipids
fats.

Glucose
a type of sugar; the chief source of energy for living organisms.

Electrolytes
chemicals in the blood that help regulate nerve and muscle function and help the body maintain its balance of fluid; examples of electrolytes are sodium, potassium, chloride, and calcium.

measure your blood chemistry before you start treatment and on a regular basis while you are receiving treatment to be sure there is no damage and that treatment is safe to give. If the blood tests show that any of your organs are not functioning normally, the doctor may decide to reduce the dose of the treatment or stop it altogether.

Some treatments can cause changes in your body chemicals, for example, lowering the magnesium level in the blood. Blood chemistries can also be affected by dehydration, which may be caused by nausea, vomiting, or diarrhea. Your doctor will also order blood chemistry tests if he or she is concerned that you may have any of these problems. If the blood tests show that certain electrolytes are too low, your doctor may decide to replace these, and if the tests show you are dehydrated, you may be given extra intravenous fluids.

It is important to have all the tests your doctor orders, because most of the time, you will not have symptoms if your blood chemistry is affected. However, sometimes people do experience symptoms such as confusion or difficulty thinking, sleepiness, fatigue, nausea, or vomiting.

> Call your doctor or nurse if you have a difficulty thinking, excessive sleepiness, or uncontrolled nausea, vomiting, or diarrhea.

80. I have heard that some people can get diabetes from their treatment. How is this diagnosed and treated?

The pancreas secretes a hormone called insulin into the bloodstream. Insulin enables glucose (a form of sugar) to be transported into your cells, giving you energy throughout the day. Normally, the pancreas adjusts the amount of insulin secreted based on what you eat and on your activity level. This keeps the level of glucose in your blood controlled at about 80 to 120 mg/dl. If your pancreas is not able to secrete an adequate amount of insulin or if your body becomes partially resistant to insulin, the glucose is not able to enter your cells effectively. As a result, the level of glucose in your blood will rise, called **hyperglycemia**. Diabetes is persistent hyperglycemia. There are a number of reasons people with cancer may develop diabetes:

- Cancer of the pancreas
- Treatment with steroids
- Family history of diabetes
- Obesity, especially with high blood pressure and abnormal blood lipid levels

Symptoms of diabetes include frequent urination, thirst, fatigue, blurred vision, and weight loss. Diabetes is diagnosed by a blood test; an elevated fasting blood glucose level indicates the presence of diabetes.

Throughout your treatment, your doctor will periodically check your blood chemistries, including the glucose level. If you develop persistent elevations in your blood glucose, you may be referred to an **endocrinologist**, a doctor who specializes in hormonal diseases, including diabetes. Additional blood tests may be ordered, and the best treatment for you will be determined. This may involve a change in diet and an increase in exercise. You may also have to take either oral medication or insulin, which is injected under your skin. The endocrinologist may also arrange to have someone teach you how to test your blood glucose levels at home.

The goal of treatment is to keep your blood glucose levels as close to the normal range as possible. This is impor-

Hyperglycemia
abnormally high blood sugar.

Diabetes is diagnosed by a blood test.

Endocrinologist
a doctor who specializes in diagnosing and treating hormone disorders.

tant to prevent long-term complications, which can result in heart and blood vessel disease, strokes, visual problems, kidney problems, and neurologic problems.

Additional information on diabetes is available from the National Diabetes Information Clearinghouse, at *diabetes.niddk.nih.gov/*.

81. What are paraneoplastic syndromes?

Paraneoplastic syndromes are believed to be caused by hormones or other substances that the tumor produces. This can cause symptoms in areas of the body at a distance from the tumor. For some people, a paraneoplastic syndrome can be the first sign leading to a diagnosis of cancer.

Paraneoplastic syndromes are rare. They occur more commonly in association with solid tumors, especially lung cancer, but they can occur with any cancer. Because paraneoplastic syndromes are caused by the tumor, treatment and control of the tumor usually results in control of the paraneoplastic syndrome.

The most common signs and symptoms of a paraneoplastic syndrome are changes in the blood chemistry (for example, high calcium, low sodium), peripheral neuropathy, joint pains, and an increased risk for blood clots. The diagnosis is made by physical examination and blood tests, x-ray, or ultrasound. Successful treatment of the cancer will usually control the paraneoplastic syndrome. Sometimes, the doctor will need to give you additional medicine to help treat the problem. It is important that you take the medicine exactly as your doctor prescribes.

PART EIGHT

Other Health–Related Issues

I get a flu shot every year. Should I get one now that I am getting treated for cancer?

Is it safe for me to be around children who have recently received a vaccine?

Should I follow up with my regular doctors while I am getting treated for cancer?

More . . .

82. I get a flu shot every year. Should I get one now that I am getting treated for cancer?

Pete's comment:

I have been getting the flu shot every year. In my case, the flu shot and pneumonia shot were administered by my oncologist. My wife also received both of these vaccinations to minimize the threat of her getting the flu and passing it on to me.

If you are getting treatment for cancer, it is important that you get a flu shot every year.

If you are getting treatment for cancer, it is important that you get a flu shot every year. Influenza is a serious disease that occurs annually. If you get influenza while you are getting treatment for cancer, it will be more difficult for your body to fight the virus and you can get very sick.

Influenza (flu) is a contagious virus that occurs every year; the peak season is usually from January through March. The most common symptoms of flu are fever, chills, cough, headache, muscle aches, and sore throat. If you get the flu you will be sick for several days, and people who have weakened immune systems may get sicker and need to be hospitalized. Even if you get the flu shot, you can still catch the flu, but getting the shot will reduce your chances of getting the flu and reduce the symptoms if you do get it.

The best time to get the flu shot is in October or November; however, you will still benefit from the shot even if you get it as late as January. You will be protected from the flu about 2 weeks after you get the shot, and this protection can last for as long as 1 year. Other members of your family should also get the flu shot to lessen their chances of getting the flu and giving it to you. Pregnant family members should check with their obstetrician before getting a flu shot.

The flu shot will not give you the flu, but it can cause some mild symptoms:

- Soreness, redness, or swelling at the injection site
- Muscle aches
- Fever

Very rare symptoms include allergic reaction and Guillain-Barré syndrome. You should not take the flu shot if you are allergic to eggs, have a history of Guillain-Barré syndrome, or have had an allergic reaction to a previous flu shot. If you are sick or have a fever when the shot is scheduled, your doctor will postpone the injection until you recover. Your doctor may also decide to postpone your vaccination if your white blood cell count is low.

There are two types of influenza vaccine. The one that has been used for many years is the "flu shot"; this is an inactivated (killed) form of the influenza virus. FluMist is a new way to get vaccinated for the flu; it is an intranasal, live, influenza vaccine. This vaccine is only approved for people ages 5 to 49 years who are healthy.

If you are getting treatment for cancer you and your family (or other household) members should not take FluMist.

For more information about the flu shot, you can contact the Centers for Disease Control and Prevention at 800-232-2522 or you can get information through the Internet at *www.cdc.gov/ncidod/diseases/flu/fluvirus.htm*.

Other Health-Related Issues

You can also get information from your local or state health department.

83. What is the pneumonia vaccine? Should I get it?

Streptococcus pneumoniae is the bacteria that causes the most common kind of pneumonia in this country, pneumococcal pneumonia. Pneumococcal pneumonia is a serious disease that causes high fever, cough, and stabbing chest pains. The pneumococcal vaccine (Pneumovax) will reduce your chances of getting pneumococcal pneumonia. This vaccine will not prevent viral pneumonia or pneumonia caused by bacteria other than *S. pneumoniae.*

If you are getting treatment for cancer, ask your doctor if you should get the pneumococcal vaccine. If you are getting treatment for Hodgkin's disease or are having a bone marrow transplant, the timing of these treatments with administration of the pneumococcal vaccine is critical; you must check with your doctor before getting the vaccine.

Unlike the flu shot which is given yearly, the pneumococcal vaccine is given once. Some people will need to be revaccinated after 5 years. If you have had the pneumococcal vaccine more than 5 years ago and you are getting treatment for cancer, ask your doctor if you need to have another vaccine.

The pneumococcal vaccine can be given at the same time as the flu shot, but it should be given in the opposite arm. You should not get the pneumococcal vaccine if you have a fever or feel sick. The vaccine can be postponed until you feel well. You should not get the vaccine if you have an allergy to any component of the vaccine. The most common reactions to the vaccine include soreness, redness, and swelling at the vaccine site; fever, muscle aches; and malaise.

For more information on the pneumococcal vaccine, you can contact the Centers for Disease Control and Prevention at 800-232-2522 or you can get information through the Internet at *www.cdc.gov/nip*. You can also get information from your local or state health department.

84. Is it safe for me to be around children who have recently received a vaccine?

In the United States, the Centers for Disease Control and Prevention (CDC) recommends a regular schedule of vaccinations for children and adolescents. The vaccination schedule starts at birth and goes up to the ages of 13 to 18 years. The recommended vaccinations include hepatitis A and B; diphtheria, tetanus, pertussis (DPT); inactivated polio (a shot); measles, mumps, rubella (MMR); varicella (chickenpox); influenza; and pneumococcal vaccine (see Questions 82 and 83 for more information).

All the above are inactivated (killed) vaccines, except for varicella and FluMist (the new inhaled influenza vaccine), which are "live" vaccines, made from weakened virus. Although rare, children (or adults) given the varicella vaccine or FluMist could transmit the disease to susceptible people.

If you are getting treatment for cancer and a member of your household has been vaccinated, check with your doctor or nurse to see if you should avoid contact with the person who was vaccinated.

Other Health-Related Issues

For more information, you can also contact the Centers for Disease Control and Prevention at 800-232-2522, or you can get information through the Internet at *www.cdc.gov/nip*. You can also get information from your local or state health department.

85. Should I follow up with my regular doctors while I am getting treated for cancer?

If you are getting treatment for cancer, you should talk to your doctor or nurse about your regular health maintenance and disease prevention routines (for example, mammogram, colonoscopy, dental care, Pap smear, PSA level, blood lipid level). You should continue your normal routine if possible; however, while you are getting your cancer therapy some of these routines need to be scheduled at a "safe" time. Other physicians that you see need to be told that you have cancer, and they need to know what treatment you are taking. For example, before making an appointment for dental work, you need to notify your oncologist and your dentist. Together they will decide when you should schedule your visit and if you need to take antibiotics or have a complete blood count before your appointment.

If you are getting treatment for cancer, the doctor taking care of you is likely a medical, surgical, or radiation oncologist, a doctor who in the last few years of his or her training specialized in the care of people with cancer. In addition to treating your cancer, your oncologist is capable of performing a complete history and physical examination, ordering and interpreting the results of tests, and prescribing medications. You will want to make sure that your oncologist shares results of his or her examinations, tests, and prescriptions with your other doctors because this may cut down on duplication of tests and extra expense for you or your insurance company.

Many people (but not all) who have cancer also have other medical problems, such as diabetes, hypertension (high blood pressure), heart disease, lung disease, and arthritis. In some cases, if your medical problem(s) is mild or well controlled, your oncologist may be able to help you manage or monitor your problem. In other circumstances, such as if you have difficult to control diabetes or heart disease, you will want to continue to see your personal physician. There is not a "right" way to handle these circumstances. This is a decision that you and your oncologist need to make together depending on the seriousness of your cancer and your other health-related problems.

How to handle other medical problems is a decision you and your oncologist need to make together.

86. Can I drink alcohol?

Lisa's comment:

I was surprised when my nurse told me there were no alcohol restrictions during chemotherapy treatment for breast cancer. However, since most of my oncology nursing experience comes from the Gastrointestinal Service (esophageal, stomach, colon, rectal, liver, and pancreatic cancers), I couldn't help but refrain from alcohol consumption. If I drank at all, it was at least a week after treatment. I had few side effects during therapy. Perhaps not drinking was key?

Recently, there has been much media attention concerning the health benefits of regular light to moderate alcohol consumption. There are reports of decreased incidence of stroke, positive effects on the heart, and other beneficial effects. Additionally, for many people, having a drink before dinner will stimulate the appetite.

Alcohol can interact with many medications, including certain treatments for cancer. This can result in intensifying the effects of some medications or making others ineffective. Additionally, even though alcohol is high in calories, high alcohol consumption can interfere with the absorption of nutrients in the stomach and small intestine. Furthermore, some antibiotics can cause severe nausea, vomiting, and headache when alcohol is consumed.

If you are getting treatment for cancer, talk to your doctor or nurse about consumption of alcohol while you are getting treatment. Depending on your circumstances, you may be able to have an occasional drink. Other doctors will recommend that you do not drink any alcohol at all.

87. Should I stop smoking?

There are no benefits to smoking tobacco.

If you smoke cigarettes or other tobacco products, you need to stop smoking. There are no benefits to smoking tobacco products. Smoking contributes to serious respiratory diseases (emphysema and chronic bronchitis), peripheral vascular disease (diseases of the blood vessels that carry blood to the arms and legs), and heart disease. In addition to causing lung cancer, smoking is also a risk factor for other cancers of the mouth (oral), voice box (larynx), bladder, kidney, pancreas, cervix, and stomach, and some types of leukemia.

If you have cancer or are getting treatment for cancer, it is important that you stop smoking. Research has shown that people with cancer who stop smoking live longer than those who do not stop smoking, even in people who have lung cancer. If you continue to smoke, you are at greater risk from side effects of surgery, chemotherapy, and radiation therapy. You are also at greater risk of developing a second type of cancer. Smoking also increases the risk of developing other diseases, such as those mentioned above.

Some people have little or no difficulty when they stop smoking; others are either unable to quit or they resume smoking at a later time. Some people are nicotine dependent and can experience withdrawal symptoms when they stop smoking. If you are currently smoking tobacco products, talk to your doctor or nurse; they can recommend strategies for quitting.

Nicotine replacement therapy, other medicines, behavioral modification, and support groups are available to help you quit smoking. A combination of all elements is used in comprehensive smoking cessation programs. Your doctor or nurse can recommend a program for you.

There are a number of nicotine replacement therapies. Nicotine gum and nicotine patch (Nicorette, Habitrol, NicoDerm CQ) are available over the counter. Nicotine inhaler and nicotine spray (Nicotrol) are available by prescription. All nicotine replacement products are associated with side effects:

- Headache
- Dizziness
- Upset stomach
- Blurred vision
- Unusual dreams or nightmares
- Diarrhea

If you continue to smoke, you are at greater risk from side effects of surgery, chemotherapy, and radiation therapy.

Other Health-Related Issues

Nicotine replacement therapy should be used with caution in people who have significant heart problems, including recent heart attack. To see if nicotine replacement therapy is safe for you, check with your doctor or nurse.

Bupropion (Zyban) is another type of medicine available by prescription that can help you to quit smoking. It was originally used as an antidepressant (called Wellbutrin), but research shows that this medicine is also helpful for people who want to quit smoking. Bupropion alone is often not enough to help people quit smoking. It is usually used in addition to nicotine replacement therapy as part of a smoking cessation program.

For more information on smoking cessation, you can contact the American Cancer Society at 800-227-2345 or on-line at *www.cancer.org*. Additional information on smoking cessation and nicotine replacement therapy can be obtained through the American Lung Association at 800-586-4872 or on-line at *www.lungusa.org*.

PART NINE

Emotional and Social Concerns

How can I better cope with having cancer?

I have completed treatment and my doctor
tells me there is no evidence of cancer. How do I
go on with my life and start feeling "normal" again?

How can I talk with family
and friends about my cancer?

Where can I get more information about cancer
symptoms and side effects of treatment?

More . . .

88. How can I better cope with having cancer?

Lisa's comment:

My ability to cope with the diagnosis of cancer probably stems from having a strong oncology knowledge base. I think I would have been more overwhelmed if I didn't know anything about cancer and its treatments. It is true, though, that too much knowledge can be a bad thing!

I am a no-nonsense type of gal. Once diagnosed, I sought the best medical care possible, had confidence in my physicians and nurses, and accepted the love and support of family and friends. I received comfort in my already active religious life and truly felt my burdens spiritually lifted.

Pete's comment:

The emotions that I went through after being told that I have lung cancer ran the gamut from anger to fear to emotional overload. I had thought of myself as a relatively healthy man who was in good physical condition. Now, I face a devastating cancer diagnosis that could dramatically affect my quality of life. I was also dejected and frustrated that I would not be able to accomplish so many things that I wanted to do. I find that by focusing on the moment and the "next right thing," I am able to keep things in perspective and prevent myself from getting out of control. I also find that by discussing options, approaches and priorities constantly with my wife, I am able to feel much more comfortable.

When confronted with any type of difficulty or stressful situation, people tend to react and cope in ways that are characteristic for them. Some people tend to turn away from what is happening and try to shut it out for a period of time, whereas others tend to face things head on. Some people are most comfortable facing difficulties alone, whereas others prefer to have the support of family or friends. Some people want to share their thoughts and feelings about the experience, whereas others are more private and prefer not to talk about how they are feeling. Some people use humor to help them face difficulties, whereas others are much more serious in their approach. Some people want detailed information about what is happening, whereas others want to hear only what they must know. Some people want to be actively involved in making all the decisions that must be made, whereas others prefer to defer the decision making to their family or to their doctor.

How have you generally responded to difficulties or solved problems in your life? What strategies do you characteristically use when faced with stressful situations? Have these worked for you in the past? Do you feel they will be effective for you in facing the challenges ahead of you now? If you feel comfortable with the strategies you have used in the past to cope and feel confident they will be effective for you now, there is no reason to think you have to change. In fact, it will be helpful to explain to your family and friends and to your doctors and nurses what coping strategies are most effective for you so they can support you in using these.

However, if you feel that your typical ways of coping may not be effective in dealing with your cancer or if you feel the challenges are too great, learning new ways of coping will help you. This is something you may be able to do on your own or with your family and friends. However, many people find it helpful to work with a professional counselor or therapist when learning new ways of coping with difficulties in their lives. Question 91 has suggestions on how to find a professional to help you.

89. I feel so many different emotions throughout the day. How can I feel more in control?

When faced with a life-threatening illness it is normal to react with many different emotions. You may find yourself denying the diagnosis at times and having difficulty acknowledging or accepting the full reality of what you are facing. You may feel anger that this is happening to you, anger at the medical establishment, anger at yourself, or even anger at God. You may feel worried about what treatment will be like and about your uncertain future. You may feel sad about the disruptions in your life, the loss of your independence, or the possible loss of all you expected to be and experience in the future. Most people with cancer experience some or all of these feelings at one time or another. At certain points in time you can expect these feelings to be especially strong. Difficult times for many people are when they are first told of the diagnosis, when they are faced with making decisions, just before they start treatment, if they find out the cancer has recurred or spread, or if they find there is no longer an effective treatment for the cancer. Do not be surprised if feelings that you thought had passed earlier come back to the surface at these times.

There is no right or wrong way to feel. Allow yourself to experience your emotions and try to understand and clarify what you are thinking and feeling.

There is no right or wrong way to feel. Trying to block your feelings or trying to control them may cause you undue distress or suffering. Instead, allow yourself to experience your emotions and try to understand and clarify what you are thinking and feeling. There are a number of ways of doing this, and a combination of strategies may work best for you:

- Reflect on what you are experiencing and try to clarify in your mind what you are thinking and feeling.
- Write your thoughts and feelings in a journal.
- Talk about your thoughts and feelings with someone you trust and feel supported by. This can be a close family member or friend, your doctor or nurse, a professional counselor or therapist, or a religious leader or pastoral counselor. Many people feel an immediate sense of relief once they have said out loud what they are feeling inside.
- Talk with other patients who have cancer and listen to how they describe their experiences.

Regardless of how you approach this, once you have recognized exactly what your thoughts and feelings are, you will be better able to clarify what it is you want and need. You can then direct your energy to getting these needs met, which will contribute to feeling more in control of the situation.

There are other strategies you can use to improve how you feel emotionally. Many people find that physical activity, even a brief walk or bike ride, enhances their feeling of well-being. Others find specific mind–body techniques to be helpful. These include such things as progressive muscle relaxation (alternately tensing and relaxing the muscles in one part of the body at a time), hypnosis, meditation, and mental imagery.

Emotional and Social Concerns

Many people feel an immediate sense of relief once they have said out loud what they are feeling inside.

90. Are there support groups where I can talk with other patients going through the same thing I am?

Support groups can provide the opportunity to be with other patients with cancer. You can share your thoughts and feelings with the group, and you can hear how other people have reacted to and dealt with the same challenges you are facing. This can be very helpful, because one of the most difficult parts of having cancer is feeling alone, that no one really understands what you are going through.

A health professional or a trained patient leader generally leads a support group. The group may be set up only for people with a particular kind of cancer, or they may be open to people with any type of cancer. They may be very structured, or they may be more social and informal. They may be very educationally focused, with speakers on different topics, or they may provide interaction and sharing of people's individual experiences. They may be just for patients, just for families, or allow both to participate. They may meet for a defined period of time with a limited membership, or they may be open ended, allowing people to come and go as they like. You should think about what would be most helpful to you when selecting a specific group.

There are increasing numbers of on-line support groups; some of these are for patients with a particular type of cancer. On-line support groups are usually not moderated by a professional, and the information you receive may not be accurate. Recommendations or advice you receive from an on-line support group should be discussed with your doctor. On-line support resources include Cancer Hope Network at *www.cancerhopenetwork.org* or 877-HOPENET and OncoChat at *www.oncochat.org*.

There are a number of ways to find out about support groups where you live or on the Internet. You can get a referral by asking your doctor or nurse; calling the department of Social Work at your local hospital; or contacting Cancer Care, the American Cancer Society, or the Cancer Information Service of the National Cancer Institute for a referral. Other programs also offer support groups:

- Gilda's Club, *www.gildasclub.org* or 888-GILDA-4-U
- Wellness Community, *www.thewellnesscommunity.org* or 888-793-WELL

91. My emotions are often overwhelming, and I feel distressed much of the time. How do I know if I need professional help? Where can I get professional help in coping with my emotional concerns or to improve my ability to cope with having cancer?

As described in Question 89, it is normal to react with many different emotions after being diagnosed with cancer. However, it is important to differentiate these normal emotional reactions from those that cause significant distress or suffering. Some signs that you are in distress are as follows:

- You are having so much difficulty accepting the reality of what is happening to you that you cannot make decisions about your care.

- You are so angry that you are not able to trust your health care providers.
- You are so worried and anxious that you find it difficult to understand and absorb the information you are getting, you are having difficulty making decisions, or you are having difficulty solving everyday problems.
- You feel anxious much of the time, with a constant feeling that something dreadful is going to happen. This may be accompanied by feeling nervous, shaky, or jittery; sweating; feeling tightness in your chest or stomach; or feeling that your heart is racing.
- You are sad and tearful throughout most of the day.
- You have become depressed and lost interest or pleasure in those aspects of your life that you previously enjoyed. This may be accompanied by feelings of despair or hopelessness or by problems with energy, sleep, appetite, or concentration.
- You find yourself unable to communicate as you usually do with your family or friends.

Addressing your emotional distress is as important as addressing any physical symptoms you are having.

If you are experiencing any of these continuously for more than 2 weeks or if your feelings become very upsetting or interfere with your daily life, discuss these symptoms with your doctor or nurse. Although this may not seem important enough to discuss with your doctor, addressing your emotional distress is as important as addressing any physical symptoms you are having. Ask your doctor or nurse about obtaining help from a mental health professional. Seeking this kind of treatment is not a sign of weakness and in fact can enhance your ability to cope. This is particularly true if you have had anxiety or depression in the past. Treatment can involve therapeutic counseling, medication, and a variety of techniques using your body and mind. These include such things as progressive muscle relaxation (alternately tensing and relaxing the muscles in one part of the body at a time), hypnosis, meditation, and mental imagery.

There are many types of professionals who can help you deal with your emotions and improve your ability to cope with having cancer. Mental health professionals include **psychiatrists, psychologists, social workers**, and psychiatric nurses. These are all licensed or certified in their specialty. They can all provide counseling, and psychiatrists and some psychiatric nurses can prescribe medication. Religious leaders, pastoral counselors, or hospital chaplains can assist you to find strength and support in the spiritual dimension of your life.

There are a number of ways of getting referrals to one of these professionals: Ask your doctor or nurse; contact your hospital's department of Social Work, department of Psychiatry, or Chaplaincy service; contact Cancer Care, the American Cancer Society, or the Cancer Information Service of the National Cancer Institute; or speak with the religious leader at your local house of worship.

92. I have completed treatment and my doctor tells me there is no evidence of cancer. How do I go on with my life and start feeling "normal" again?

Lisa's comment:

I never felt so loved before than when being diagnosed with cancer. I received well wishes, telephone calls, visits, flowers, get well cards and mass cards from everyone in various aspects of my life. And, yes, my relationship with

Emotional and Social Concerns

Psychiatrists

doctors who specialize in the prevention, diagnosis, and treatment of mental illness; a psychiatrist can prescribe medicine.

Psychologists

specialists who can talk with patients and their families about emotional and personal matters, and can help them make decisions.

Social workers

professionals who are trained to talk with people and their families about emotional or physical needs, and to find them support services.

family and friends have been enhanced and enriched. I didn't think it was possible.

Completing treatment for cancer brings its own set of challenges. Among these are adjusting to changes in your body, recovering strength after treatment, resuming your usual activities, returning to work, and explaining your illness to friends and colleagues. Each of these presents a new hurdle to overcome. Give yourself time and remember to draw on your usual methods of coping as well as those that are newly learned as you transition into feeling "normal" again (see Question 88).

Despite the fact that your treatment is over, you will probably find it difficult at times to balance the hopefulness that the disease will not come back with the knowledge that the future is always uncertain. Maintain a schedule of regular follow-up visits with your doctor and have blood tests and scans periodically to evaluate how you are doing. Many people find that the days immediately before their doctor's appointments and the days waiting for the results of diagnostic tests are times of anxiety and worry.

Three resources will be particularly helpful to you as you adjust to your life as a cancer survivor:

1. *Facing Forward, A Guide for Cancer Survivors*, published by the National Cancer Institute, describes the experiences of other survivors, provides practical suggestions on specific topics, and lists resources for more detailed information.
2. The Cancer Survivors Network of the American Cancer Center, at *www.acscsn.org*, offers recorded discussions on particular issues and provides an opportunity to interact with other survivors.

3. The National Coalition for Cancer Survivorship, at *www.canceradvocacy.org/*, is an advocacy organization for cancer survivors. The website contains information, practical tools, and links to resources for cancer survivors.

Despite the fears and uncertainties that lie ahead, some people find that having been diagnosed with cancer has provided them the opportunity to think about their lives in new ways. Relationships often become stronger and are enriched by the experience. And sometimes, people choose to shift the priorities in their life, ensuring they are spending their time doing what is most important to them.

DEALING WITH FRIENDS, FAMILY, AND WORK

93. How can I talk with family and friends about my cancer?

Lisa's comment:

During the early stages of my diagnosis and surgical plans, I remember getting fed up repeating myself to various friends or talking incessantly about my treatment plan or cancer in general. I would finally say: "Could we please change the subject!" I am not one to dwell on things or to be "fussed" over, and cancer did not change that aspect of my personality!

For some people, having cancer is a lonely experience. However, for others it is a time of feeling closely connected with friends and family. Being able to talk with others about your cancer can make an enormous difference in how you experience this challenging time in your life. It can help to overcome the feeling that you are alone, and it provides others the opportunity to offer you their help and support. However, you may not be ready to share your thoughts and feelings right away, and over time you may want to share certain feelings but keep others private.

If family or friends are pressuring you to speak about this before you are ready, tell the person that you appreciate their concern but that you are just not ready to talk yet. Don't push them away; reassure them that you will speak with them when you are ready. When you do actually tell people about what is happening, you will probably find that being direct and honest is the easiest approach. Some people even find it helpful beforehand to rehearse what they will say.

You will probably find that being direct and honest is the easiest approach.

You may find that some friends or family members will be uncomfortable hearing about your diagnosis. They may pull away from you, not calling or visiting as they used to. This is probably because of their own fears and anxieties about cancer or because they do not know what to say to you. Consider how important this person is to you. If it is someone you don't care very much about, there is no reason to spend any time or energy trying to reach out. However, if this is someone whose relationship you value, you may want to call them and directly express to them that you miss them. Tell them that you wish you could speak to them or see them more often, and ask if there is anything you can do to make it easier for them. This may break the ice and allow them to feel more comfortable. However, you will still find that some people will disappoint you. On the other hand, there will be people who will surprise you in their willingness to be helpful and supportive of you.

94. How can I talk with children about my cancer?

It is a common reaction to try to protect children from the news that a family member has cancer for fear of frightening or upsetting them. However, children can always sense when something is wrong at home. It is much better for them to hear directly from you about what is happening rather than overhearing something by accident or imagining something worse.

Children will cope best when they are informed. Set aside time to talk with them as soon as possible after you have been diagnosed and be open and honest when you speak with them. You may want to include the following information:

Children will cope best when they are informed.

- The fact that you are sick and that you have cancer
- The type of treatment that is planned
- If you will need to be in the hospital for a period of time
- The likely side effects of treatment and how they will affect how you look and what you will be able to do

When speaking with children, select language that is appropriate to their age and ability to understand. You might find it helpful to practice what you want to say before you sit down with them. After you have spoken with them, encourage the children to ask questions and check to see that they understand what you have told them. However, be aware that they may only be able to hear so much at a time. You may need to break down the information and address only one or two topics at a time when you speak with them.

Emotional and Social Concerns

The children may ask if you will die, or they may ask for reassurance that you will get better. Respond to their questions as honestly as you can. If you have been diagnosed with cancer at an early stage with a high probability of cure, it will be easier to reassure them. However, if you have advanced disease and they ask if you will die, you might want to explain that some people die from cancer and that the doctor is not sure right now if they can make the cancer go away. Tell them that you are hoping you will be okay and that the doctor is doing everything he or she can to help you. If they ask you when your treatment will be over, if you will be receiving treatment for a defined period of time, tell them the planned date. However, it is okay to tell them you don't know. Reassure them that as things change you will tell them what is happening.

Describe to the children how your disease and treatment will affect them. Explain who will take care of them if you will be in the hospital or if you will be coming home late from doctors' visits or treatments. Explain how their usual routines and activities may be affected. Be sure to ask them if there is anything in particular they are worried about.

There are a number of resources available to help you speak with children about cancer and to help them cope with your diagnosis:

- The American Cancer Society has several resources. On the website, in the section, "Talking About Cancer—Talking with Family and Friends," there are sections specifically addressing children. They also publish books on the topic, *Our Mom Has Cancer, Because . . . Someone I Love Has Cancer*, and *Cancer in the Family: Helping Children Cope with a Parent's Illness.*

- The National Cancer Institute publishes *When Someone in Your Family has Cancer* for young people who have a parent or other family member with cancer.
- Pottersfield Press through Nimbus Publishing offers *When a Parent is Sick: Helping Parents Explain Serious Illness to Children,* by Joan Hamilton (ISBN 895-900-40-9), 800-NIMBUS-9 (800-646-2879).
- University of Michigan Health System lists additional resources at *www.cancer.med.umich.edu/learn/pwtalking.htm*
- KidsCope is a website designed to help children understand and deal with the effects of cancer on a parent and is at *www.kidscope.org.*

95. Should I work during my treatment? Should I tell my supervisor and coworkers about my diagnosis? What if I don't feel well enough to work?

Lisa's comment:

I felt compelled to share my diagnosis with my colleagues almost immediately. I work in an oncology setting. I wanted to openly discuss my hopes and desires, fears and concerns. I felt my absence from work affected them, so they deserved to know why I would not be around for a while. I also didn't want my colleagues to feel like they couldn't talk to me about my disease and treatment. I didn't want to be uncomfortable with my life changes, and therefore they wouldn't be uncomfortable either. After surgery and my first cycle of chemotherapy, I returned to work. I felt a need for normalcy and I wanted to help with staffing. My supervisor and co-workers were tremendously supportive and truthfully helped me through the chemotherapy and radiation treatments.

Emotional and Social Concerns

If you feel productive and energized by your work or if you enjoy the camaraderie you experience at work, you will probably want to continue working during your treatment if you are able. Many people feel quite well during cancer treatment and can continue working, either full time or part time. However, other people do not feel well enough to work or must make accommodations in their hours of work or in the specific functions they do at work. Tell your doctor or nurse about the type of work you do and your usual hours of work. Ask them how they expect you to feel during treatment and what they recommend in regard to your continuing to work.

People who continue to work often feel unsure whether to tell anyone about their situation, whom to tell, and how much to tell. Some people want to talk openly about their diagnosis and treatment with colleagues whose support helps them cope with treatment. Other people are more private and prefer that people at work not know about their situation. Some people are even afraid they will be treated differently, that they will be discriminated against, or that they may even lose their job if people at work know they are ill.

The Americans with Disabilities Act protects people who are disabled from being discriminated against at work. It requires employers to make reasonable accommodations as long as you can perform the essential functions of your job. However, people unfortunately do not always respond the way we hope they will or that the law requires. You may find that your supervisor believes you will not be able to perform as well on the job, and you may lose the opportunity to work on certain projects or even to be promoted. You may find that your coworkers will be uncomfortable hearing about your diagnosis. They may pull away from you, not talking with you as they used to. This is probably because of their own fears and anxieties about cancer or because they do not know what to say to you. Some coworkers may even worry that they will have to do more work because of your illness, which may make them resentful.

If you need accommodations in the type of work you do or in the hours you work, you must speak with your supervisor about the situation. Prepare ahead for this conversation. First, consider how you can get the most important parts of your job done. Then determine how you need to alter the hours you work to balance getting the job done with taking care of your medical needs. Being open with your supervisor from the beginning can be extremely helpful. He or she can guide you in obtaining information about your rights and your benefits and can work with you to make the accommodations you need and to make adjustments over time as your needs change. If you find it difficult to speak directly with your supervisor about this, speak with someone in the human resources department. If you have a conflict with your supervisor and human resources is not able to help, you may need to contact an attorney for guidance.

You can contact the following for more information about the Americans with Disabilities Act and how it applies to you:

- United States Department of Justice, at *www.usdoj.gov/crt/ada/adahom1.htm* or by phone at 800-514-0301
- United States Equal Employment Opportunity Commission, at *www.eeoc.gov/* or by phone at 800-669-4000

Speak with your supervisor or someone in the human resources department about your options.

If you are unable to work or must change to part time work, speak with your supervisor or someone in the human resources department about your options. Find out about your disability benefits. Be aware that the Family and Medical Leave Act allows eligible employees up to a total of 12 weeks of unpaid leave during any 12-month period. For information about this, contact the human resources department where you work or the United States Department of Labor at *www.dol.gov/esa/whd/fmla/*.

Cancer and Careers at *cancerandcareers.org* is a valuable resource for people with cancer, their employers, and their coworkers. It addresses all these issues and provides helpful tips and suggestions from other patients about living and working with cancer.

FOR FAMILY AND FRIENDS

96. How can I help, and what is the right thing to say?

It is often difficult to know how best to help someone you care about who has been diagnosed with cancer. There is no answer to this question that is right for everyone. Match what you are able to do and would like to do with the specific things that person needs.

Try to anticipate what they will need and make specific offers.

You may find it easiest to start with concrete things. However, a general offer of "let me know if I can help with anything" is not the best approach. This requires the person to think about what he or she needs and then ask you for help. Instead, try to anticipate what the person will need and make specific offers. Plan these for days when you know the person may need more help than usual, like days of doctor's visits or treatment or when they are feeling particularly ill or tired. The possibilities are unlimited, but here are a few examples of things you might be able to offer:

- Drive them to a doctor's visit or treatment
- Drop off a cooked dinner for the family
- Spend a morning cleaning the house
- Launder the family clothes
- Shop for food and needed household items
- Invite the children for a sleepover
- Arrange to pick up or meet the children after school

Another way of helping is to offer your presence. Would the person appreciate company because they live alone or while the rest of the family is working or at school? Offer to visit and bring lunch, to accompany them for a walk, to bring a video you can both watch, to go out shopping together, or to have them come spend the weekend with you. Again, the possibilities are unlimited. The key is to match what you are able to do and would like to do with the specific things they enjoy. One word of caution, however: This person may not have the energy to participate in many of the things you used to do together. Consider how they are feeling at the time and don't create unrealistic expectations for them. You may need to plan short visits. Make the time together pleasurable regardless of what you do or how long you spend together.

It is natural to feel unsure of the right things to say when someone you care about has been diagnosed with cancer, is undergoing difficult treatment, or perhaps is facing the end of their life. You may feel afraid to ask the person how they are doing because you are nervous you will not know how to respond to their answers. You may feel concerned that if you say the wrong thing you

Emotional and Social Concerns

193

will hurt them. You may feel worried that if you talk about your own sadness, or even cry, you will cause the person distress. Because of your own discomfort, you may try to withdraw from the situation, distancing yourself from the person, calling less often, and putting off visits. This can result in leaving the person feeling abandoned and alone at a time when they need your presence in their life more than ever before.

There is no script you can follow as a guide in knowing what to say. In fact, if you make assumptions about what the person is thinking or feeling, you may unintentionally say things that will cause distress. The best way to start is by listening. Let the person know that if they would like to talk about their illness you would like to listen. At the same time, remember that not everyone communicates in the same way. Some people are very open and want to share everything they are thinking and feeling with those they are close to. Others are more private and prefer not to talk about these things. Even for people who are generally more communicative, there may be times they feel like talking and other times when they do not want to. The important thing is to let the person know you are available to listen and to let them control when and how much they choose to share. If they want to speak with you of their thoughts and feelings, the greatest gift you can give is to be present and to listen.

The greatest gift you can give is to be present and to listen.

However, listening to things that are painful to hear about or being with someone who is emotionally distressed or crying may be uncomfortable for you. You may find yourself wanting to change the subject or even offering reassurances that everything will be okay, even if that may not necessarily be true. Although this may help in dealing with your own discomfort as the listener, it does not help the person speaking. In addition, it may give the message that you do not really want to hear what they have to say. Try to overcome your own discomfort and remain present to hear what they are saying. It is okay to tell the person that this is difficult for you and that you are not sure how to respond to what they are saying.

It is okay to tell the person that this is difficult for you and that you are not sure how to respond.

You also may want to speak to the person who is ill about thoughts or feelings you are having. You may want to tell them how much you love and care about them. You may want to tell them of your own sadness or feelings of helplessness. You may want to try to reconcile if you have previously had a conflict. You may want to speak with them of your own worries and concerns related to their illness. We often leave a great deal unsaid in an attempt to protect those we love. Yet in fact it is the unsaid things that are often the most important things to say.

97. At times I feel that the responsibility of caring for this person is very difficult. Do other people experience similar feelings?

When someone is diagnosed with cancer, there are numerous stresses and demands placed on family and friends. These stresses will be greatly influenced by the person who is ill: their age, the role they play in the family, how advanced the disease is, the type of treatment they are getting, the symptoms they are experiencing, how physically disabled they are, and how they are emotionally responding to their illness. Regardless of the individual situation, there are several sources of stress for those who are providing care.

Emotional and Social Concerns

One demand placed on caregivers is the need to provide physical care to the person who is ill. The past 20 years have brought many changes in health care. One of the most significant is that many people who were previously cared for in the hospital are now cared for at home. This places the responsibility of providing physical care on family and friends. This includes ensuring the person is comfortable; administering medications; managing equipment and supplies; observing for relevant signs or symptoms; knowing when to call the doctor or nurse; and, if the person is very ill, helping with bathing, dressing, feeding, moving, and walking. If the person has advanced disease, these demands will increase if the person gets sicker.

Another demand placed on caregivers is the need to address the nonmedical aspects of care. These include scheduling and coordinating appointments, providing transportation, obtaining medications, running errands, supervising others who may be providing care, as well as handling medical bills and other financial matters. In addition, there are numerous decisions to be made every day and the need to solve problems that regularly arise.

Making this even more difficult is the fact that when you become a caregiver your usual day-to-day responsibilities don't just go away, and you may also have to take on those responsibilities previously handled by the person who is now ill. Further complicating things for some people is that based on the relationship they have previously had with the person who is ill, they may have ambivalent feelings about the fact that they now need to take care of them.

All the stresses and demands placed on you as a caregiver can lead you to feel overwhelmed at times. You may become exhausted or even physically ill. In addition, you may find yourself experiencing a variety of difficult emotions: anger, guilt, fear, and sadness. Finding ways of caring for yourself, attending to your physical and emotional needs, and using the resources available to you can help you effectively attend to the needs of the person who is ill while making this experience a positive and meaningful one for you. Question 98 lists resources available to help caregivers succeed in this role.

Finding ways to care for yourself can help you attend to the needs of the person who is ill.

98. How can I get help so that I can provide support and care to this person without being overwhelmed by the demands?

The physical and emotional demands of caregiving are significant. The first step to getting help is to acknowledge how this is affecting you and identify which demands are the greatest for you. Are you having difficulty in regard to the time needed for care: visiting in the hospital, accompanying the person to doctor's visits or treatment, having to do more at home, or needing to take time off of work? Are you having difficulty in regard to the finances needed for care: inadequate medical insurance for doctor's visits and treatments, expensive medications, costs of travel, costs of missed work time, costs of extra services you need to pay for, like extra babysitting? Are you having difficulty in regard to the physical burdens of providing care if the person is weak and debilitated: needing to assist with walking or lifting, needing to bathe and feed, needing to administer medications, perhaps needing to move in with them for a period of time? Are you having difficulty with the overall responsibility of managing their

Emotional and Social Concerns

197

medical care when you don't feel you have adequate knowledge or skills to do this effectively?

You can take several approaches to help you manage the demands you may be experiencing as a caregiver. Most important is to ensure you have the information you need to feel capable of providing care. Schedule time to speak with the person's doctor or nurse in the office or over the phone to review the plan of care and discuss issues of concern you have. Some specific questions you may want to ask are as follows:

• What is the goal of treatment?
• What do you expect will be the outcome of the treatment?
• What side effects may occur from the treatment?
• How can the side effects be managed?
• What medications have been prescribed? What are they for? What dose should be given and at what times of the day?
• What are reasons I should call your office?

Ask if they have any written material to give you that reinforces the information they have reviewed with you.

To manage the many things that must be done each day, divide the work.

To manage the many things that must be done each day, divide the work. Identify among family members and friends who is able and willing to do what part of the work. However, remember that people do not always respond the way you want them to respond. Families that generally work well together at times of stress will work well together in providing care. However, families in which there is a previous history of disagreement may find it difficult to overcome patterns of conflict. Furthermore, each member of the family will have a different idea about what they can manage. This may not match your own expectations. Based on each person's ability and willingness, assign a schedule for each person to do the different tasks needed.

If you need more assistance at home than family or friends can provide, ask your doctor or nurse if they can refer you to a social worker to explore what home care services are available to supplement what the family can provide. These services include visits by a registered nurse to provide skilled nursing care (for example, changing a dressing, giving an injection), home health aides to assist with personal care (for example, bathing or being present in the home to assist the person during hours your are not available), and homemakers to assist with tasks at home (for example, cooking, cleaning, and laundry). You will need to verify with the person's health insurance company what services are covered. If there is no coverage for help at home, consider if you or other members of the family have the financial resources to pay for these services.

There are other resources that may be helpful in providing support to you as a caregiver. Educational programs designed specifically for caregivers of people with cancer may be available in your community. You can find out about these through the American Cancer Society, the Cancer Information Service of the National Cancer Institute, Cancer Care, or the department of Social Work at your local hospital. There are other good resources:

• National Family Caregivers Association at *www. nfcacares.org* or 800-896-3650. Be sure to view the section entitled "Most Frequently Asked Questions."

- National Coalition for Cancer Survivorship at *canceradvocacy.org*. The Cancer Survival Toolbox includes a section entitled "Caring for the Caregiver."
- Family Care America at *www.familycareamerica.com*.
- *Caregiving: A Step-By-Step Resource for Caring for the Person with Cancer at Home*, published by the American Cancer Society.

Combat the isolation many caregivers feel by reaching out to people who can support you.

Key to being able to provide care to someone else is to also find ways of taking care of your own needs. Combat the isolation many caregivers feel by reaching out to people who can support you; spend time with them and talk about how things are going. Schedule time for yourself to do things you enjoy, like taking a walk, listening to music, or reading a book. Don't try to do everything yourself; divide the work and let others help.

Caregiving is stressful and has many demands. It can be seen as a burden, or it can be seen as an opportunity. In caring for another person, you may learn of inner strengths that you never knew you had, you may find you are more competent and capable than you had previously realized, and you may feel spiritually enriched. Family and friends may come together with a renewed sense of purpose and connection. And finally, caregiving provides you the opportunity to express your love for that person in the most intimate way imaginable.

99. How do we manage the financial burdens cancer places on our family?

When a person is diagnosed and treated for cancer, the financial burdens placed on the family are enormous. The patient may not be able to deal with the many financial issues that must be addressed, so many people find it helpful if a particular family member or friend takes over this responsibility. There are a number of steps that will be helpful with this.

Review the patient's health care benefits thoroughly to determine exactly what they are entitled to. Many policies are confusing, and if you are not clear on the benefits, speak with someone in the human resources department where the person works or contact the insurance company directly. There are specific questions you may want to ask:

- Can any doctor treat the person, or must they use someone in the health plan? How much more will you have to pay if they use a doctor outside the plan ("out of network")?
- Does the plan include coverage for a second opinion?
- Do they need authorization before having particular diagnostic tests or treatments? What is the process for obtaining this?
- Does the plan cover care only at particular hospitals?
- Does the plan provide home care only with particular agencies?
- Does the plan include coverage for prescription medications?

Meet with a financial counselor where the person will be receiving treatment to determine the estimated costs of care. Work with them to calculate what you have to pay out of pocket based on the person's insurance coverage. If you will not be able to pay this, discuss how you can work out a payment plan that will be realistic for you.

If paying for care will be difficult, meet with a social worker to find out what financial assistance is available. The person may be entitled to government or charitable assistance. The American Cancer Society and Cancer Care may also be able to provide financial assistance.

The cost of prescription medications can be significant. Many pharmaceutical companies have assistance programs to provide medication at a reduced cost. To find out about financial assistance available for particular medications, ask the nurse or social worker for information. Resources that list pharmaceutical companies with assistance programs are as follows:

- Cancer Care at *www.cancercare.org*, under Helping Hand Guide select "Drug Assistance Programs"
- Pharmaceutical Research and Manufacturers of America (PhRMA) at *helpinghands.org*
- NeedyMeds at *www.needymeds.com* or (215) 625-9609

Transportation is another area in which the financial costs can quickly mount. Speak with a social worker to get information about transportation services in the region. Cancer Care and the American Cancer Society can also provide information and may be able to offer limited financial assistance for transportation.

Track all the financial costs incurred related to the disease and treatment. Speak with an accountant when the person is first diagnosed to learn what is tax deductible and what records you should keep. The following costs are tax deductible for many people:

- Medical costs not covered by insurance. These include annual deductible costs, co-pays (the fees that are paid up front for specific services), and co-insurance (the

part of the bill the insurance company doesn't cover).
Keep copies of all bills and claim forms.

- Expenses paid to maintain the person's health insurance policy.
- Out-of-pocket expenses, including those paid for prescription medications and transportation to medical appointments. Keep mileage records and receipts for all of these.

100. Where can I get more information about cancer symptoms and side effects of treatment?

The Internet is increasingly becoming the most up-to-date source of comprehensive information on cancer and cancer treatment. If you do not have a computer of your own, ask a family member or friend if you can spend time using their computer. Most local libraries also have computers available to use for free, and hospitals are increasingly making computers available for their patients to use.

Most of the Internet addresses we have listed in the Appendix that follows will bring you to the home page of each organization. Although specific areas of the site may be pointed out, spend time searching within each site to find the information you are looking for as well as to explore the other information and links you come across. Your time will be rewarded as you increase your knowledge and understanding of your disease and treatment and as you discover the numerous resources for information and support that are available to help you, your family, and friends.

Tips for managing cancer symptoms and side effects of treatment are found on many of the sites listed.

Emotional and Social Concerns

Additional sites are mentioned within questions addressing particular symptoms or side effects. We recommend that you speak with your doctor or nurse before trying anything recommended on the Internet.

Search engine
a program(s) on the internet that helps you find information on topics of interest; examples include yahoo and google.

Internet addresses often change over time. Those listed in the Appendix are all accurate as of March 2004. If you cannot find the organization at the address listed, try using a **search engine** to find it. Telephone numbers are also listed if they are available.

American Cancer Society (ACS)
Coping with Treatment section addresses symptoms and side effects.
Internet: *www.cancer.org*
Telephone: 800-ACS-2345

Association of Cancer Online Resources
A collection of cancer-related Internet sites.
Internet: *www.acor.org*

CancerCare
Focuses on providing information for emotional support and practical help.
Internet: *www.cancercare.org*
Telephone: 800-813-HOPE (4673)

Cancer Information Network (CancerLinksUSA)
Provides information and links to other cancer-related sites.
Internet: *www.thecancer.info*

CancerSource
Section for patients includes information on symptom management.
Internet: *cancersource.com*

Cancer Survivors Network
Sponsored by the American Cancer Society, provides a forum for communicating
with other cancer survivors; also has a listing of resources.
Internet: *www.acscsn.org*

National Cancer Institute (NCI)
Publications addressing symptoms and side effects that are particularly helpful in-
clude the following:
Chemotherapy and You: A Guide to Self Help During Treatment
Radiation Therapy and You: A Guide to Self Help During Treatment
Eating Hints for Cancer Patients
Pain Control: A Guide for People with Cancer and Their Families
Advanced Cancer: Living Each Day

When Cancer Recurs: Meeting the Challenge
Internet: *cancer.gov*
Telephone 800-4-CANCER (Cancer Information Service)

National Coalition for Cancer Survivorship

Among the useful resources is The Cancer Survival Toolbox.
Internet: *www.canceradvocacy.org* (under Programs, select Cancer
   Survivor Toolbox, an audio program on coping)
Telephone: 877-NCCS-YES

National Comprehensive Cancer Network (NCCN)

Has guidelines for managing specific symptoms, including pain,
   fatigue, nausea and vomiting, and neutropenia (low white blood
   cell count).
Internet: *www.nccn.org*
Phone: 888-909-NCCN

Oncolink

Sponsored by the University of Pennsylvania, the Coping with
   Cancer section addresses symptoms and side effects.
Internet: *www.oncolink.com*

Oncology Nursing Society

Provides information on managing fatigue, anorexia (loss of appetite), pain, depression, neutropenia (low white blood cell
   count), and cognitive dysfunction.
Internet: *cancersymptoms.org*

People Living with Cancer

Sponsored by the American Society of Clinical Oncology
   (ASCO); has a section on Managing Side Effects.
Internet: *www.peoplelivingwithcancer.org*
Telephone: 703-797-1914

Steve Dunn's Cancer Guide

Provides information on many cancer-related topics.
Internet: *www.cancerguide.org*

Some published resources may also be useful to you:

Caring for the Patient with Cancer at Home, A Guide for Patients and Families
American Cancer Society, 2001

Choices
Marion Morra and Eve Potts
HarperCollins, 2003

Living Well With Cancer: A Nurse Tells You Everything You Need to Know About Managing the Side Effects of your Treatment
Katen Moore and Libby Schmais
Perigee Trade, 2002

Managing the Side Effects of Chemotherapy and Radiation Therapy
Marylin J. Dodd
UCSF Nursing Press, 2001
Order from University of California San Francisco, 415-476-4992

Glossary

Acupuncture: a technique of inserting thin needles into the body at specific locations with the goal of restoring the normal flow of energy in the body; often used to treat pain or other symptoms.

Addiction: an uncontrollable psychological craving for a substance such as a drug or alcohol.

Adjuvant chemotherapy: treatment used after a tumor has been removed surgically to destroy any remaining cancer cells.

Advance directives: legal documents in which you indicate who you want to make medical decisions for you and/or what type of medical care you want to receive if you become unable to make decisions or speak for yourself.

Analgesics: medications to treat pain.

Anemia: a condition in which the number of red blood cells is below normal.

Antiemetics: medication used to prevent or treat nausea and vomiting.

Antihistamine: medication that is used to prevent or treat allergic reactions; it is sometimes given to treat itching caused by a rash.

Ascites: abnormal build up of fluid in the abdominal cavity.

Benign: a non-cancerous tumor; can expand and press on surrounding structures, but does not invade surrounding structures and cannot spread to a distant site.

Biologic therapy: treatment to stimulate the immune system to destroy cancer cells, make the cancer cells more vulnerable to being destroyed by the body's own immune system, or strengthen the ability of the immune system to destroy the cancer cells; also called biotherapy, biologic response modifier therapy, and immunotherapy.

Botanicals: plants or plant parts valued for their medicinal properties; includes herbal products; commonly prepared as a tea, an extract, or a tincture.

Brachytherapy: radiation treatment that involves the placement of sealed radioactive material (for example seeds or wires) into the body where they emit radiation as they decay (break down); also called implants or internal radiation.

Catheter: a thin flexible tube that is used to administer fluid into the body or to drain fluid from the body.

Cerebral edema: swelling of the brain from inflammation or other diseases.

Chemotherapy: treatment with drugs that destroy cancer cells or stop them from growing.

Clinical trials: research studies to test the effectiveness of new treatments on human beings.

Cognitive dysfunction: difficulty remembering names, places, or events or trouble with language skills, concentration, or arithmetic.

Combined modality therapy: the use of a combination of treatments to destroy cancer cells.

Complete blood count (CBC): a blood test to measure the number of white blood cells, red blood cells, and platelets.

Computed tomography (CT): a diagnostic test that creates images of structures in the body using x-rays and a computer; slices or cuts of the body in a particular area can be seen.

Consent form: a written document signed by a patient to indicate that they have been informed about a particular treatment and of the risks and benefits associated with that treatment and agree to receive the treatment; also referred to as "informed consent."

Cystitis: inflammation or irritation of the bladder.

Diuretic: a medication that increases the production of urine; also called a "water pill."

Do not resuscitate (DNR) order: indication in a patient's medical chart based on the expressed wishes of the patient or their health care proxy that no extraordinary life-extending measures are to be taken if they stop breathing or if their heart stops beating.

Doppler ultrasound: a procedure in which high-energy sound waves (ultrasound) are bounced off internal tissues or organs and make echoes that form a picture of body tissues called a sonogram; used to determine if there is a blood clot in a blood vessel in an arm or leg.

Dosimetrist: a member of the radiation oncology team who designs treatment plans and calculates the dose of radiation the tissues will receive when treated with radiation therapy; works in collaboration with a medical physicist and a radiation oncologist.

Dyspareunia: pain or discomfort during sexual intercourse.

Dyspnea: difficult or labored breathing; shortness of breath.

Dysuria: pain or burning on urination; usually caused by irritation or infection of the bladder or urinary tract.

Electrolytes: chemicals in the blood that help regulate nerve and muscle function and help the body maintain its balance of fluid; examples of electrolytes are sodium, potassium, chloride, and calcium.

Eligibility criteria: list of conditions that must be met for someone to enroll in a clinical trial.

Emboli: blood clots that travel through blood vessels and eventually obstruct or block the flow of blood.

Endocrinologist: a doctor who specializes in diagnosing and treating hormone disorders.

Endometriosis: a benign condition in which tissue similar to that which lines the uterus grows in abnormal places in the abdomen.

Epidermal growth factor (EGF) receptor: protein found on the surface of some cells; when EGF binds to the protein receptor it stimulates the cell to divide.

Extravasation: a potential complication of intravenous chemotherapy administration that occurs when chemotherapy leaks from the vein into the surrounding tissue.

Feeding tube: a tube placed through the abdominal wall into the stomach; this is used to give liquid nutritional supplements.

Fluid retention: a condition in which the body does not eliminate adequate fluid and can cause swelling and weight gain.

Glucose: a type of sugar; the chief source of energy for living organisms.

Grade: a measure of how abnormal a cell appears when examined under a microscope; in some cases predicts how aggressive the cancer.

Guided imagery: a technique in which patients use their imagination to visualize something they desire, for example visualizing the chemotherapy attacking their cancer cells.

Health care proxy: a person designated to make health care decisions for you if you are not able to; also called a health care surrogate, a medical proxy, or a medical power of attorney.

Hematocrit: the proportion of blood which is red blood cells; expressed as a percentage; used as a measure of the amount of red blood cells.

Hemoglobin: substance in red blood cells that binds to oxygen and carries it to the tissues of the body; used as a measure of the amount of red blood cells.

Hemoptysis: spitting up blood or blood-tinged sputum.

Homeopathic medicine: treatment with extremely small doses of substances that produce symptoms of illness in healthy people when given in larger doses to stimulate the body's own healing responses.

Hormonal therapy: treatment that alters specific hormone levels in the body by stopping the production of the hormone, blocking the hormone, or adding hormone.

Hospice: a program that provides care to patients at the end of their life; can be provided at home or at an inpatient facility.

Hyperglycemia: abnormally high blood sugar.

Incontinence: urinary incontinence is the uncontrolled loss or leakage of urine.

Inferior vena cava filter: the inferior vena cava is a large vein that empties into the heart and carries blood from the legs and feet and from organs in the abdomen and pelvis; a filter (umbrella-like device) may be placed in the inferior vena cava to prevent blood clots in the legs from traveling to the lungs.

Intensity-modulated radiation therapy: a method of planning and delivering radiation therapy that uses 3-dimensional images of the body to precisely aim multiple beams of radiation with varying intensities to the target tissue from many different angles; this minimizes the dose received by the surrounding normal tissues.

Internist: a physician who specializes in the diagnosis and medical treatment of adults.

Intraoperative radiation: the administration of radiation to the tumor site during surgery.

Jaundice: yellowing of the skin and the whites of the eyes resulting from buildup of bilirubin in the tissues; can occur if the bile ducts are blocked or if the liver is not functioning; accompanied by darkening of the urine and lightening of the color of the stools.

Kegel exercises: exercises designed to increase muscle strength and elasticity in the pelvis; may be recommended for treatment of urinary incontinence.

Linear accelerator: a machine that uses electricity to create high-energy radiation.

Lipids: fats.

Living will: document in which you can state specific instructions regarding your health care, including measures that would prolong your life; may outline which medical interventions you want to have performed and which you want to have withheld for a variety of circumstances.

Locally advanced: describes when a cancerous tumor has spread to surrounding structures.

Lymph nodes: bean-shaped structures in the lymphatic system that filter lymph fluid before it is returned to the blood stream.

Lymphedema: a condition in which lymph fluid collects in tissues after removal or damage to lymph nodes, from surgery or radiation therapy; usually occurs in an arm or leg.

Macrobiotic diet: a diet that consists of whole grains and cereals that may be supplemented with beans and vegetables; varies in how restrictive it is and may not provide adequate nutrients.

Magnetic resonance imaging (MRI): a diagnostic test that creates images of structures in the body using radio waves and a powerful magnet.

Malignant: a cancerous tumor; can invade surrounding structures and spread to a distant site.

Metabolism: a series of chemical reactions in which cells convert nutrients to energy.

Metastasized: describes when a cancerous tumor has spread to a distant site, for example the bones, the liver, or the brain.

Mucous membranes: thin tissues that line many of the cavities and passageways of the body, for example the gastrointestinal tract, the respiratory tract, and the genitourinary tract.

Myalgias: aches and pains in the muscles.

Naturopathic medicine: use of a variety of interventions (for example, dietary modifications, massage, exercise, acupuncture) based on the belief they can enhance the body's natural healing forces.

Neoadjuvant chemotherapy: treatment with chemotherapy before the primary treatment, for example before surgery; often used to shrink the tumor.

Nerve block: a procedure in which alcohol or a local anesthetic is injected into or around a nerve to treat pain.

Nerve-sparing surgery: a surgical procedure for men with prostate cancer in which the prostate is surgically removed and the nerves are left undisturbed with the goal of maintaining erectile function.

Neurologist: a physician who takes care of people who have problems or diseases of the nervous system.

Neutropenia: A decrease in the number of neutrophils, the type of white blood cell that fights infection and other diseases.

Neutrophils: A type of white blood cell that fights infection and other diseases.

Nocturia: frequent urination that occurs at night.

Obstruction: blockage in a passageway.

Oncologist: a physician who specializes in treating cancer; surgical oncologists specialize in cancer surgery; medical oncologists specialize in treatment with chemotherapy, hormonal therapy, and biologic therapy; radiation oncologists specialize in treating with radiation.

Orthomolecular: treatment with specific doses of vitamins, amino acids, fatty acids, trace minerals, electrolytes, and other natural substances based on the belief that disease may be cured by restoring the optimum amounts of substances normally present in the body.

Osteoporosis: a condition that is characterized by a decrease in bone mass and density (thinning of the bones), causing bones to become fragile.

Palliation: relief of symptoms; palliative care (supportive care) refers to treatment aimed at relieving physical, emotional, social, and spiritual symptoms to improve quality of life.

Paracentesis: a procedure in which a thin needle or tube is placed through the abdominal wall to remove fluid from the peritoneal cavity.

Glossary

213

Paraneoplastic syndrome: a group of symptoms that may develop when substances released by some cancer cells disrupt the normal function of cells and tissue away from the tumor; it can be a cause of cognitive dysfunction.

Peripheral neuropathy: a condition of the nervous system that causes numbness, tingling, burning or weakness; usually begins in the hands or feet and can be caused by certain anticancer drugs.

Peritoneal cavity: the space within the abdomen that contains the intestines, stomach, and the liver; lined by thin membranes.

Platelets: blood cells that help prevent bleeding by causing clots to form when a blood vessel is cut; also called thrombocytes.

Pleural effusion: abnormal build up of fluid in the chest cavity.

Pleural space: the pleura are membranes that line the inside of the chest wall and cover the outside of the lungs; the space between the membranes is called the pleural space.

Pleurodesis: a medical procedure that uses chemicals or drugs to cause inflammation and adhesion between the layers of the pleura (the tissue that covers the lungs and lines the interior wall of the chest cavity) to prevent the buildup of fluid in the pleural cavity; used as a treatment for severe pleural effusion.

Positron emission tomography (PET): a diagnostic test that creates images of the body based on metabolic activity; radioactive glucose (sugar) is injected and because cancer cells have a higher metabolic rate than normal cells, the glucose will go to those cells and become visible on the scan.

Postherpetic neuralgia: localized pain that occurs in the area where shingles was present.

Prostate gland: a gland within the male reproductive system that is located just below the bladder surrounding part of the urethra, the canal that empties the bladder; produces a fluid that forms part of semen.

Prostatitis: inflammation or infection of the prostate gland.

Pruritus: itching.

Psychiatrists: doctors who specialize in the prevention, diagnosis, and treatment of mental illness; a psychiatrist can prescribe medicine.

Psychologists: specialists who can talk with patients and their families about emotional and personal matters, and can help them make decisions.

Pulmonary embolism: a blood clot in the lung. A pulmonary embolism usually starts when a blood clot travels from a vein in the legs to the pulmonary artery; this can cause sudden shortness of breath.

Radiation therapy: the use of high-energy radiation to destroy cancer cells; also called radiotherapy or irradiation.

Radioactive isotopes: unstable elements that emit radioactivity as they decay (break down); used to take diagnostic images or to treat cancer.

Radionuclide scanning: a diagnostic test that creates images of the body; after radioactive material is injected or swallowed it collects in particular organs of the body; a scanner creates an image based on measurements of radioactivity in the organ.

Red blood cells: cells in the blood that contain hemoglobin that carries oxygen from the lungs to all the tissues in the body; also called erythrocytes.

Reiki: a technique of hands-on touching based on the belief that this touching channels the body's spiritual energy which leads to spiritual and physical healing.

Remission: a disappearance of all signs and symptoms of cancer; cancer cells may still be in the body.

Search engine: a program(s) on the internet that helps you find information on topics of interest; examples include Yahoo and Google.

Shunt: implantation or creation of a permanent tube to move blood or other fluid from one part of the body to another part; for example, to control ascites, sometimes a shunt is placed in the abdomen to direct the fluid into the bloodstream.

Social workers: professionals who are trained to talk with people and their families about emotional or physical needs, and to find them support services.

Stage: a measure of how extensive the cancer is, how much it has spread.

Stereotactic radiosurgery: a method of delivering multiple precisely defined beams of radiation to a small area of the brain in a single treatment.

Steroids: medications that are used to relieve swelling and inflammation; in people with cancer, steroids can be used to help other problems such as nausea and vomiting, pain, breathing and loss of energy.

Stomatitis: inflammation or irritation of the mucous membranes in the mouth; this can be caused by chemotherapy or radiation therapy.

Thoracentesis: removal of fluid from the pleural cavity through a needle inserted between the ribs.

Three-dimensional conformal radiation therapy: a method of planning and delivering radiation therapy that uses 3-dimensional images of the body to precisely aim multiple beams of radiation to the target tissue from different angles; this minimizes the dose received by the surrounding normal tissues.

Thrombosis: the formation or presence of a blood clot inside a blood vessel.

Topical anesthetic: medication applied to the surface of the body (for example the skin or mucous membranes) to numb the area.

Tumor: an abnormal swelling or mass.

Urologist: a doctor who specializes in problems or diseases of the urinary tract.

Vesicants: chemotherapy that causes blistering or other local tissue damage if it leaks from a vein into the surrounding tissue. Only some types of chemotherapy are classified as vesicants.

White blood cells: cells in the blood that fight off infection and other types of disease; also called leukocytes; there are many different types of white blood cells that include neutrophils and lymphocytes.

Index

Index

Index